LION
UNLEASHED

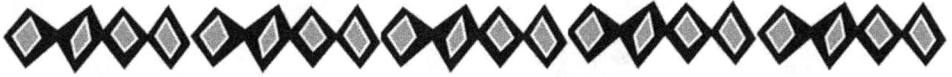

LION UNLEASHED
A JOURNEY OF WEIGHT LOST AND COURAGE FOUND

by

Stephen Hosaflook

What Readers Are Saying About
LION UNLEASHED

"I had the opportunity to work with Steve for twelve weeks teaching and educating him on how to change his LIFESTYLE, something a diet didn't do. The most important thing I teach and the one thing Steve has now learned...It ALL starts with the FORK!"

~ Butch "Mr. Wellness" Temnick, MFCS, CHS, CLC

"I really enjoyed reading Steve's *Lion Unleashed*. The story of his journey to physical fitness is honest, funny, thoughtful, realistic, and inspiring."

~ Jennifer Myers - Jen's Total Fitness, Warren, Ohio

"I loved Lion Unleashed! Funny, motivational, educational, revealing. Steve is the 'real deal' when it comes to getting results with weight loss. Don't waste time with fad diets. Read this book...and read it again! He tells you the truth about what it takes and how exactly to do it. *Lion Unleashed* is a must read for anyone trying to lose weight and keep it off."

~ Dr. John Mistretta - Back to Health Chiropractic, Warren, Ohio

"*Lion Unleashed* is an excellent source of fitness and fat loss information for anyone and everyone ready for permanent lifestyle change. He really has an uncanny ability to get inside your head and to help you think your way to a healthier and happier life. I cannot think of a better leader by example."

~ Darin Steen - Personal trainer, author of *The Fatloss Lifestyle*
12 Week Body Transformation Program, and owner of Steen's
Elite Physique's Training Studio, Chicago, Illinios

"As a coach and athletic director at the scholastic and college level for over 30 years, I believe Steve Hosaflook's weight loss is the finest physical, mental and spiritual accomplishment I have personally witnessed. Now the world will see what I have always known that Steve is truly a "Lion." More importantly, this book is not about self-reliance but understanding who you are and what God, through Christ, can do in your life if you are willing to let Him."

~ Bruce Johnson Baseball Coach Grove City College

Copyright

Copyright © 2010 by Stephen Hosaflook

1st Paperback Edition

ISBN-13: 978-1-934561-20-1

Printed in the United States of America

Submit requests for reprint permission
to the publisher at:

Vidi Press
11721 Whittier Blvd. #203
Whittier, CA 90601
800-409-7170
service@vidipress.com
vidipress.com

DEDICATION

◆◈◈◈

*I dedicate this book and my golden years
to helping my millions of brothers and sisters
overcome our common foe—obesity.*

ACKNOWLEDGMENTS

My heart is filled with great joy and gratitude for all the people mentioned below and others not mentioned who have guided, pulled, pushed, insulted, and encouraged me on this journey…and will continue to do so. I know I couldn't have pulled it off and I won't be able to "keep it off" without them. From the bottom of my heart, thank you all.

First and foremost, I want to give a big thank you to my Lord and Savior, Jesus Christ who has been with me every step of the way. I am incomplete and nothing without Him. All praise and thanks to You, my Lord.

My mom and dad have been in my corner my whole life and have been a huge motivational influence on me. How can I fail when I see them battling ongoing illnesses every single day? Thank you, Mom and Dad. My love for you is boundless.

Thanks to Dr. John Flauto at the Warren Foot Clinic who diagnosed me with the heel spur and Achilles tendonitis that started this big ball rolling. No heel spur, no story.

Thank you to all the great folks at TuDor Physical Therapy Centers. If I had not found this special place I don't know where I'd be today. The list of those I want to thank is long so I'll begin with the founders and owners, Sam and Laura Dye. Thanks to your vision this special place has improved and lengthened countless lives. A special thanks goes to the "full of life" Tina Amorganos, for her great contributions to this book. And I want to thank "super stud" Dan Sharfal who helped me better understand weight training. They both helped me more than they'll ever know. One other big thank you goes to Julie Rhodes. She did the majority of the physical therapy on my knee after the arthroscopic surgery but I think she missed her true calling…a fighter in the MMA (Mixed Martial Arts). I call her the "submission hold" expert because she made me "Tap Out". (In other words, she made me give up…while bending me like a pretzel.) Many thanks also to Dana Smith, Jeanine Spangler, Tori Schuette, and D.J. Nutt. I appreciate all their kind words and ongoing encouragement and count them all as friends.

I owe a debt of gratitude to Joyce Ringold who has been and will forever be a great source of inspiration to me; an incredible woman with an incredible story. Please share your story with the whole world, Joyce; the process will heal you and touch everyone who reads it.

I want to thank my cousin Alan Hosaflook who not only helped me face down two of my fears but also contributed a great deal to this book, as did his two co-workers…Phyllis Middlebrook and Kristine Jekutis.

Thanks to my good friends at Global Health and Fitness: Bill Myers, Eric Bergman, and Ahlam Buss. They willingly invested their time in me whenever I asked and they have my undying gratitude. They are amazingly kind and gifted people and Global will always hold a special place in my heart.

A special thanks to my sister Pamela Johnson who took all the photos that appear in the book.

Most recently, thank you Butch Temnick, a good Christian man who happens to be a former Mr. South Carolina body builder and has taken on the role of my own lifestyle coach. Oh yes, and he's one of the most enthusiastic people I've ever met.

I'd also like to thank Tristine Rainer whose book, *Your Life as Story* inspired me to write this book. At least, that's what really motivated me to try.

And last, but certainly not least, I want to thank Kelly Kovacic. To put it simply, Kelly saved my life, or at least dramatically transformed the quality of my life. Just how do you properly thank someone for doing that? I wish I knew. I do know this; I owe Kelly a debt I'll never be able to repay. God's providence brought her into my life. Had she not shown me how to radically change my lifestyle, I would never have experienced the joy and happiness I benefit from today. Most people go through life not knowing the impact they've had on others, but I won't let that happen to Kelly. I've heard it said that it takes a minute to meet someone special, an hour to like them, a day to love them, and a lifetime to forget them. It will truly take a lifetime for me to forget Kelly Kovacic.

TABLE OF CONTENTS

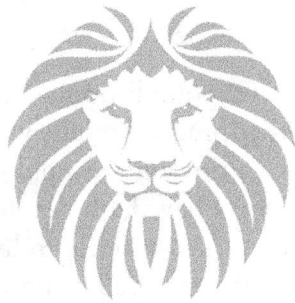

THIS LION FEELS YOUR PAIN

◇◆◇◆◇

I'm an evening custodian in a public middle school. I clean for a living. I'm just an ordinary guy who accomplished a remarkable transformation—so remarkable that I had to write about it. In fact, I want to shout about it—shout loudly enough that the whole world can hear!

Not long ago, I was fifty years old and close to retirement but hauling around 160 pounds of excess cargo prevented me from enjoying the fruits of my labor. I was destined to live my golden years as a functional invalid.

As someone once said, "If you do what you always did, you'll get what you always got." That *was* me—a yo-yo-yo dieter with no goals and no courage to commit to anything or anyone. Three times I transformed my body into a lean and mean fighting machine, but after each loss I only got bigger and bigger. Then one day I stopped doing what I always did and got something totally different than what I always got. I got a new body, a new attitude, and a new life. I now wake up every day with my eyes open like never before. I had a physical and spiritual re-awakening, if you will, that manifests itself in my new vocation—to help you fight and win your own personal battle with obesity.

You're not alone in your battle. The same failures, struggles, and challenges you face, I have faced. I'm not going to give you pie-in-the-sky psychology or patented Hosaflook diet strategies. My motivation is not monetary. I won't endorse any particular diet or exercise program. As a matter of fact, this book isn't about diets or dieting at all—at least not in the sense that most people think about diets. You see, a diet is something that starts and stops. What I've undergone in the span of one year and what I'm recommending to you is not a temporary fix, but a permanent solution.

I'm not a doctor, so I'm not licensed to give medical advice. I'm not a registered dietician, a clinical nutritionist, or a certified fitness trainer. I'm just going to tell you how I lost 160 pounds over sixteen months using good old-fashioned American values that produce results whether you're Thomas Jefferson trying to free a country or a fifty-one year old janitor trying to free himself from his blubbery confinement. I have faith that if I could do it, so can you.

An old Roman proverb says, "It is better to live one day as a lion, than a thousand days as a lamb." I can't ever recall being a lion or even lion-like when I weighed 355 pounds, but today I know that I'm going to accomplish great things as the190-pound king of my own jungle. The lion within me has finally been unleashed and this book is my roar.

PART ONE

◆◢◣◥

HOW I GOT FAT AND STAYED FAT

*To say that obesity is caused by merely consuming too many calories
is like saying that the only cause of the American
Revolution was the Boston Tea Party.*

~ Adelle Davis

1

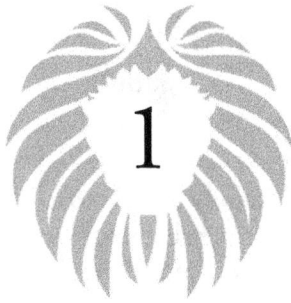

ENDURING DECEPTION

*All experience hath shown that mankind is more disposed to suffer
and endure evil than to right themselves by abolishing it.*

~ Adapted from the Declaration of Independence

◇◆◇◆

When you're hauling around 160 pounds of excess cargo all day every day, people are going to notice. Some will tell you the flat-out truth because it's their job, like my orthopedist who said, "Steve, if you don't lose 150 pounds, you could spend the rest of your life in a wheelchair!" Others will tell you the truth because they haven't yet learned they're not supposed to, like my niece, Rebecka, who climbed up on my lap, poked me in my Pillsbury Dough Boy belly and said, "Oh my gosh, Uncle Steve, you have bigger boobies than my mommy!" Certainly not what any manly ego wants to hear. Others will tell you the truth because they have never seen you before and will never see you again, like the unhelpful fellows I met on a recent golf excursion to Myrtle Beach, South Carolina.

Halfway there, my three buddies and I stopped at Krispy Kreme. We had skipped dessert after a dinner of country fried steak, mashed potatoes and gravy, green beans, and rolls, so those two-dozen glazed donuts sure hit the spot.

Before turning in for the night, we headed to a nearby movie theater for some entertainment and, of course, more goodies: "Here come four guys who are definitely ice cream eaters! How about some buy-one, get-one-free coupons, guys?" a spotty-faced theater attendant shouted as he passed out coupons outside the box office.

My brother-in-law and best friend since grade school, Bruce (weighing a mere 250 pounds) admitted, "There's a wake-up call, fellas."

"Yeah, we know we're big, but did he have to advertise it?" said Tom (who weighs in at 280 pounds).

3

We chocked it up to the kid's youthful arrogance as we proceeded to put those ice cream coupons to good use.

On day two, our trip coordinator, Derrick, met us at Myrtle Beach. It was his duty to warn us of local customs that could limit our enjoyment, so he gave us this courtesy reminder: "I can tell by looking at you guys that you're quite the beer drinkers; but remember fellas, it's Sunday and all the bars are closed around here."

Dan (a real comrade at 320 pounds) replied in a rather offended manner: "What do you mean by that? None of us drink!"

Well, Derrick kept his cool and continued to call it like he saw it: "Sorry guys, my mistake…an honest one though." Again, we chocked it up to youthful arrogance.

It was almost tee-time on day three. No sooner did our shoes hit the pavement at the Golf Club parking lot than we heard: "Holy crap! When you guys got out of that minivan, it rose a good foot and a half. It sure took a beating coming all the way from Ohio!"

I finally had enough. "Okay, that's it!" I said to my buddies. "That's the third shot about our weight in three days and I'm fed up! He gets no tip, guys!"

Tom agreed, "That's right. No tip for him!"

Well, the attendant heard our little discussion and defended himself, "Sorry guys. I just call 'em like I see 'em."

Times like these really made me appreciate my buddies. You see, whenever I asked them if I looked as big as that really obese guy across the green, they would simply say, "No Steve, you carry your weight very well." Now that's what I call compassion. Why couldn't these employees who are paid to serve us be as compassionate as my buddies?

I have an answer: discrimination and rudeness against obese people are alive and well in America. This country has come a long way in adapting to the needs of the disabled, but obesity is not protected by the Americans with Disability Act. And, I'm glad it's not or else the government would be enabling me to remain morbidly fat.

On the other hand, I'd like to enact an American PHAT ACT—**P**reventing **H**ostility **A**gainst **T**ubbiness. I closed my eyes and ears to a lot of hostility in the past, but now I see and hear it clearly. Even my cousin recently admitted that he reluctantly asked me to fly with him because of my two-seater size. I didn't understand that kind of bias until he finally invited me on my very first plane ride.

While sitting comfortably in one seat at 190 pounds, I noticed that passengers looked at large people differently. You know what I mean…that look of "Oh No! I have to sit beside him?" Or a roll of the eyes when a large woman asked for something to eat. And when an obese person went to the restroom, heads shook.

I wanted to stand up and give those rude people a piece of my mind or maybe enforce the statutes of my PHAT Act and require the offended party to sit next to the offender. Guilt would be hard to prove, however, because no one had actually said a word. I could just sense what they were thinking by the little occurrences that caught my eye.

On the ground, people feel freer to express their private thoughts about fat people. I remember stepping inside a fast-food restaurant where I saw the cashier turn to the burger flippers and say, "Better drop some more fries, there's a big guy coming!" He didn't know I heard him, but I did. Let me tell you, I didn't disappoint him either. *I'll show him*, I thought. I told him to make me a fresh sandwich! That always ticks them off. But what did I show him? That's right. I showed him that I was exactly what he saw—a big fat guy that the restaurant would make a ton of money off of.

Now that I'm thin and trim, attitudes have dramatically changed. When I ask for assistance in stores, the clerks actually help me without the snickers or off-the-cuff comments, like "Go find it yourself, fatso!" or "Maybe if you got away from the feeding trough, you big hog, you could get around a little better!"

I have to say that I never personally heard such blatant insults, but friends and relatives have told me they overhead comments like these once I was out of earshot. It took losing all of that weight to see and hear the truth of what strangers thought of me. I just didn't notice…or maybe I did notice, but I buried the truth of it like a dog buries a bone.

Have you heard the old saying: "There are none so blind as those who will not see?" That was me. I wouldn't acknowledge how grotesquely huge I was. I got angry at others for pointing it out and ignored the destruction that 160 pounds of excess fat was doing to my joints and organs. Every step I took wore away more cartilage in my knees to where bone was rubbing against bone. I even grew new bone on the back of my right heel while the tendons around my ankle screamed *Please stop!* They were terrified that I was going to rip them apart and rightly so. People warned that I could develop high cholesterol, high blood pressure, and diabetes; but fortunately as a janitor, I was quite active at work and at home as a caretaker for my parents. Had I been a couch potato all day long, I truly believe I would be dead by now.

So why did I choose to endure physical pain and social humiliation rather than acknowledge the truth and take the advice of doctors, family, and friends? And more importantly, how did I rid myself of this self-deception and regain control of my body and my life? I'll start to answer these questions by first sharing with you how I became one very soft American.

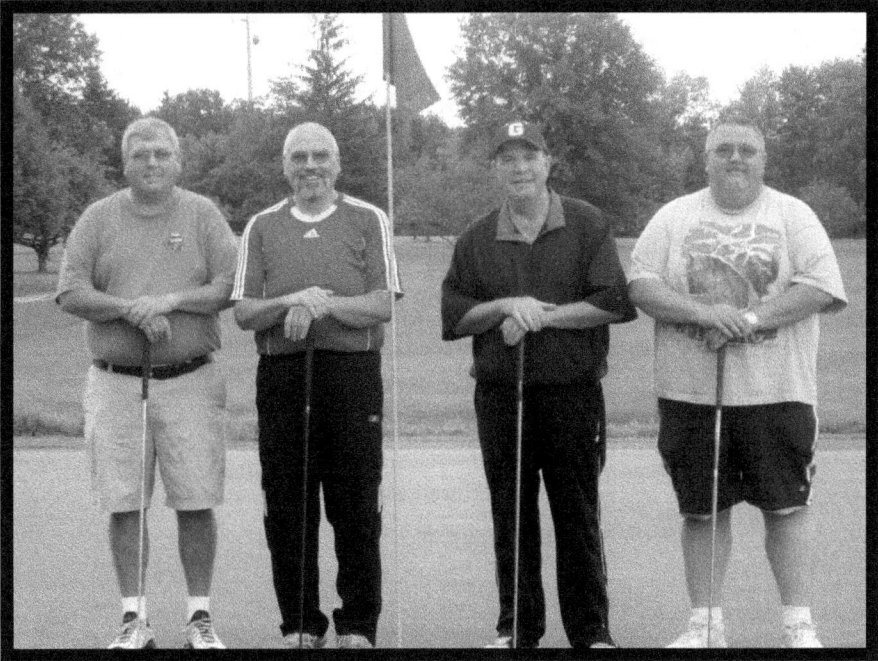

The Van Droppers: Tom Johnson, Me, Bruce Johnson, Dan Johnson

2

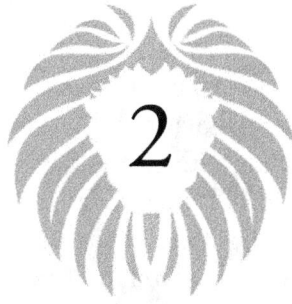

ONE VERY SOFT AMERICAN

Our struggles against aggressors throughout our history have been won on the playgrounds and corner lots and fields of America. Thus, in a very real and immediate sense, our growing softness, our increasing lack of physical fitness, is a menace to our security.

~ *The Soft American, by John F. Kennedy in Sports Illustrated, 1960*

❖◆◆❖

I was three years old in 1960 and on my way to becoming the hard American that my president would have been proud of. I was an active child, always playing ball, building tree houses, or riding my bike, constantly on the go. So what happened? Probably the same thing that happened to you in one way or another.

At age ten, I started playing Little League Baseball and was a pretty good third-baseman. By the time I was twelve, I made the All-Star team. We fell one game short of going to the Little League World Series in Williamsport, PA. When I turned thirteen, I was so looking forward to becoming a third-baseman in the Pony League (the next level up). There was no question in my mind that I would make the team and earn the position I wanted. After all, I was an All-Star.

During the six-month hiatus between leagues, I began junior high where my mom's packed-with-love lunches were no longer cool. I was a big boy now with a big boy lunch allowance. The joys of the cafeteria captured both my tummy and my money. My mom had no idea how much junk food I ate that was disguised as lunch and sold as candy. The more junk I ate, the lazier I got. By now gym class was nothing more than a mental exercise where I learned to perform just enough to get by. I didn't train for the upcoming tryouts either. I gained weight so gradually that no one seemed to notice, except when it came time to perform.

9

I showed up for the Pony League try-outs the next spring believing that I was still in my twelve-year old, All-Star body, but of course, I wasn't. I huffed and puffed around the bases, straining with great inflexibility to field ground balls. I just couldn't cover as much ground as I used to. What else is a competent coach supposed to do but look me straight in the eye and say, "Steve, I'm picking someone else to play third base. He's faster than you, he'll steal more bases for me, and cover more ground at third than you can. You were really good last year, but you've lost several steps over the winter and it cost you the position."

Now other kids might have worked hard to regain the coach's confidence, but not me. I quit. My best friend, Bruce, gave it to me straight, though: "Listen, Hoss, you made the biggest mistake of your life by quitting that team! You have no one to blame but yourself for getting fat and out of shape."

I just yelled back, "Don't ever call me that again. I'm not some big, dumb Hoss!"

In its own way, that exchange set the stage for decades of self-protecting, blaming others, and denying reality.

On the day I quit, I not only squashed any dreams of earning a paycheck by playing baseball, I also broke my dad's heart. You see, his first love was baseball. In his youth, he played for a team in the Warren AA League and a traveling team in his West Virginia hometown. He hit legendary homeruns in our tri-state area and was a natural at every position he played. One summer weekend, the old St. Louis Browns came to town looking for new talent. He didn't know it at the time, but the player they specifically came to see was my dad. Unfortunately, that weekend his family had called him to come home to care for his mom, so he missed his shot at the big leagues. He badly wanted me to become what he couldn't.

By giving up, I let him down big time. I wanted my dad to be proud of me, but I wholeheartedly believed I was a great ball player and no Pony-League coach could convince me otherwise. Yes, I was upset at losing the third-base position and disappointing my dad, but even that didn't motivate me enough to get into shape for next season's tryouts. Instead I ate more garbage, became less active, and got bigger and softer.

You would think that since I was larger than my classmates, I would have been a more powerful American kid, more able to fight those aggressors on the playground that President Kennedy warned about; but instead, I lost wrestling matches to kids who were much smaller than I was because they were in better physical condition.

Before age thirteen, my skill and speed earned me the status of first pick by the team captain during gym class. After age thirteen, my softness and slowness earned me close to last pick. I wanted to play; but to be honest, I just wasn't willing to work for it. My cousin said to me, "Steve, if only I had your skill to go along with my desire, I could've played in the NFL!"

You see, I pretty much wasted the physical talents God gave me and let down the guys at school big time. They counted on me to contribute to the team; but instead, I weighed them down with Ding Dongs and Twinkies.

I should mention that during my teen years, I played on my church's softball and basketball teams. I even played some golf, but I ate far too many double-double cheeseburgers and banana splits for that to matter. Walking around a golf course and running down a basketball court didn't burn as many calories as I ate, so I continued to gain weight.

By the age of eighteen, I weighed 225 pounds. That would be a normal weight for a seven-foot man, but I was six feet tall, which made me at least fifty pounds overweight. Worse than that, I became bigger, softer, weaker, and slower every day. Fifteen years after President Kennedy inspired a nation to make exercise a priority for the sake of national security, I (and the rest of the nation) took little interest in championing physical fitness.

Is this the shape of things to come?

It can be—with modern conveniences and push buttons. Easy living is sapping the strength and vitality of our children. One-third of them of school age can't pass minimum physical achievement tests.

Urge your school to offer at least 15 minutes of daily, vigorous activity. This can bring our nation's youth up to sound physical standards.

For a free booklet to help you evaluate the youth fitness program of your school, just write: President's Council on Physical Fitness, Washington 25, D.C.

Physical Fitness Advertisement (courtesy jfklibrary.org)

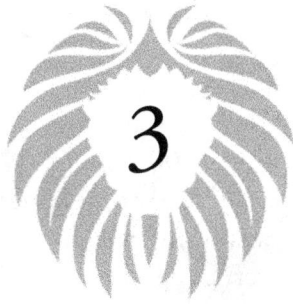

3

YO YO YO

*If you want something you have never had
you must do something you have never done.*

~ Thor Winston

By the age of twenty-two, I was pretty fat, but I didn't feel fat. In fact, I was hired as the assistant coach of a junior high football team where I taught young boys how to have self-discipline, even though it was obvious that at 285 pounds, I had none. No one actually said I was a hypocrite, but clearly it was time to practice what I preached. I started a quick-fix weight-loss program known as Atkins and darned if it didn't work. Starving my body of carbohydrates got rid of 100 pounds in a mere seven months! Now weighing in at 185 pounds, I was once again lean, mean, and setting a great example for my team—until football season ended. Then I celebrated.

For three years I partied hard, downloading pizza, potato chips, and two-liter bottles of anything with sugar. And oh, the bread! Did I ever pack that away—good old-fashioned, enriched, white bread! I didn't care or even give much thought to hypocrisy and self-discipline. All I could think about was what flavor of ice cream I would buy on the way home from work.

How much do you think I weighed after three years of this self-indulgence? No, not 285 pounds like before Atkins. I actually beat that and topped out at a whopping 300 pounds. It even sounds big doesn't it? *Three hundred pounds—* a number that screams, *Hey Steve, you might have a problem!* Through it all, I really didn't feel fat and I probably would have stayed fat if it weren't for those darn videotapes.

As the coach of the junior varsity boys' basketball team, I had to analyze our games. There I was, watching myself lead fit and fast boys and thinking

Holy cow! That's embarrassing. I've got to do something because I look disgusting!
So back on the Atkins diet I went. I was getting pretty good at this. Over the
next eight months, I lost another 100 pounds. What a success story I was—
lean and mean at 200 pounds and ready to reward myself again. I even remember thinking all the while I was losing weight: *I've been depriving myself for
too long. When this diet is over, I'm going to eat.* Brilliant!

So how long do you think it took to weigh 300 pounds again? Gradually,
it took four years. At the age of twenty-nine, I had regained every pound I had
worked so hard to lose. I was now coaching middle-school basketball where
all the other coaches boasted a lean 195 pounds just as I had twice before. But
now I was gigantic.

This is it! One final time. For crying out loud. I've done this before!
I told myself. So I created a new diet incorporating Atkins principles and darn
if it didn't work once more! Eight months later, at the age of thirty, I weighed
in at 195 pounds! What a success I was!

If I could have continued on an Atkins diet every day, then perhaps I
would have stayed at 195 pounds, but denying my body of carbohydrates long
term would have been very dangerous. Atkins does have a maintenance plan,
but that plan still limits the intake of carbs, which in turn limits the nutrients
that carbs provide. And the truth is that any diet that limits a certain food
group while encouraging other food groups creates a chemical imbalance in
both the body and the brain.

The purpose of interfering with the body's natural processes is to trick the
brain into believing you're not hungry. But if I had continued to mess with my
today's natural processes, I could have developed high cholesterol, heart disease,
diabetes, a stroke, and who knows what else. Hey, those sound just like the risks
of obesity, don't they? Well, that's because they are. Overeating and fasting mess
with the natural functioning of the body. A healthy weight-loss plan works with
the body the way God designed it to function, not against it.

My motivation to lose weight during each yo of my yo yo yo should have been
sufficient to keep the weight off. I wanted to set a good example for the kids and
look good on video and in pictures standing next to the other coaches. But down
deep, I really yearned for a sense of well-being and control that I found only while
eating. So by my mid-thirties, I stopped the yo-yo-yoing and allowed the inner me
to become everything he thought he could be—that is, 355 pounds, the biggest I'd
ever been, and more depressed than I can ever remember being.

4

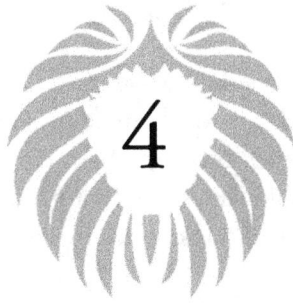

CONTROLLING FOOD CONTROLLING ME

To enjoy freedom, we have to control ourselves.
~ Virginia Woolf

During my mid-forties I became a full-time caregiver for my parents. Most caregivers have no idea how to create emotional and physical boundaries, and neither did I. We willingly sacrifice our independence, our goals, and our lives for the care of another. It's like being a missionary in your own home. No dating … No career aspirations … No thinking about your needs because if you do, the needs of those you care for will go unmet.

Every day for years, I have watched my mom battle the confines of her walker and wheelchair while coping with the pain of advanced arthritis. Every day, I've watched my dad's mental and emotional abilities fail a little more than the day before as the early stages of dementia took root. Every day I watched them deteriorate while I did for them what they could no longer do for themselves. Every day, I did a little more than the day before, and every day further depleted my emotional energy.

Friends asked why I took on so much responsibility, especially when I had my own physical problems. Colleagues wondered why my brother and sisters didn't lend a helping hand more often so I could pay more attention to my own needs. I wondered that, too, at times, but I now understand that the troubles of my siblings far outweighed my own. None of them could make the kind of commitment necessary to be a caregiver the way I could.

I was single, and I had made a vow to myself and to God to care for my parents. I needed to be needed, and I was. I became the rock of the family, the deliverer, and the problem solver: "Steve will take care of it. He's the oldest. He'll handle everything," they'd say. But I was not a rock. In fact, there were times I felt like a railroad conductor watching his train about to collide, powerless to stop it. I love my mom and dad and would care for them all over again, but I am only one man. There were times when I just felt used up. As loony as it sounds, eating helped me feel in control. After all, I could sure show that pizza who was boss! Then one day, food showed me who really held the keys to my fate.

Fat and Bone

Bone rubbing against bone hurts a lot. It throbs. It grinds. It crunches. But through it all, I continued to clean one classroom after another until one day I couldn't take one more step. The pain was so excruciating that I left work in the middle of my shift. No amount of Ibuprofen could relieve the pain enough to sleep, so I lay awake all night resolving to go to the doctor the next day, something I rarely ever do. The doc gave me a shot of that miracle drug, Cortisone, to help relieve the pain as well as a good dose of truth to try to save my life.

Apparently, the cartilage in the knee, which is designed to create a cushion between the bones in the knee joint, had worn away after decades of abuse causing osteoarthritis in both knees. I was on the fast track to becoming a disabled custodian—not a prized possession in the workforce, especially in a school building with three floors and no elevator.

As I ascended the steps, so did the pain. Dragging myself and my trash can from room to room wasn't much easier. My supervisors offered me the option of going on disability leave and I'm sure I would have qualified, but disability was not an option I could live with in all good conscience. I knew many people who continued to work while suffering more pain than I had. Instead, I started a fourth Atkins diet, but I soon lost interest because I didn't really want to diet. I wanted to eat.

Food became Cortisone to my soul. In spite of the now obvious consequences I ate even more than before—outrageous amounts of junk food. A typical day started around 8 a.m. with two Egg McMuffins, two hash browns, a cinnamon roll, and a large Coke that I called a "breakfast soda." Then about two hours later, I ate a bowl of sweet cereal and two toasted cheese sandwiches. I washed that down with a couple of cans of Coke. Two hours later I stopped at Wendy's on my way to work to get a double burger, large fries, and a large root beer. My co-worker and I would typically share an extra large pizza for lunch. She always ate two pieces I ate the rest. During the evening at work, I visited the kitchen several times to munch on cookies, cakes, pies, chips, basically anything I could find.

At 10:00 p.m., I left work. Of course, I stopped at the store on the way home to buy ice cream, potato chips, and a soda, which I ate as I watched television. I was quite comfy using my right hand to eat out of the half-gallon ice cream carton sitting on my lap and drinking from the two-liter bottle of soda with my left, setting it down only long enough to stuff down a handful of chips. I usually consumed the entire store-run in one sitting! That's got to be between 15,000-25,000 calories in one twenty-four-hour period. Unfortunately, I only burned about 5,000 calories in that same time frame, so it wasn't strange for me to consume between 10,000-20,000 excess calories—not every day, but many days.

I was in charge of what and how much I ate. That's what I called control. Nothing was off limits. If I wasn't at work or caring for my parents, I was eating or lying around the house, preferably doing both at the same time. Everyone saw it happening, including my oldest nephew J.D. who told me plainly, "Uncle Steve, if you don't do something about your weight, you're not going to be around much longer!" Of course he was right, but I just gave a great big belly laugh. You know how the world loves a guy in XXL sweatpants and XXXL shirts who laughs his way through life.

Golf Got Me Good

At least I could still enjoy golf. Shortly after my nephew prophesied my demise, I decided to play nine holes by myself in ninety-five degree weather without a golf cart. That's right. I vowed to walk the course like normal people do. However, the truth broke that vow after only six holes. With every agonizing step toward the parking lot, I prayed, "Lord, let me make it back to the car ... and please let the air conditioning work." Those 1,000 yards seemed like an eternity as I huffed and puffed the whole way.

Drenched in sweat like a hog on butchering day, I finally reached the car. I just sat inside for forty-five minutes with the engine on, air blasting, thinking, *I'm going to die ... and when that happens, who's going to take care of Mom and Dad?* Now you know how much I love my parents. I couldn't leave them, but even that thought wasn't enough to change anything. The words rushing around in my mind continued to deceive me as I thought some more: *I'm fifty-two years old. I weigh 355 pounds. My heel is killing me. My knees are shot. I can't play golf anymore. My family and closest friends can't shame me enough to fix it. For crying out loud, a doctor can't even shake me up enough! I've lost weight three other times and failed to keep it off. I guess this is the way it's supposed to be. I am what I am and I'll just have to accept it.*

So, what did I do after that little talk with myself? I stopped at Wendy's on the way home and ate my cares away. I decided to stay fat, but I could no longer take the pain of being fat. My heel was killing me. I couldn't play golf anymore. But what was worse, I could barely keep my job. God knew I was at the end of my rope physically and emotionally. That's when He took over.

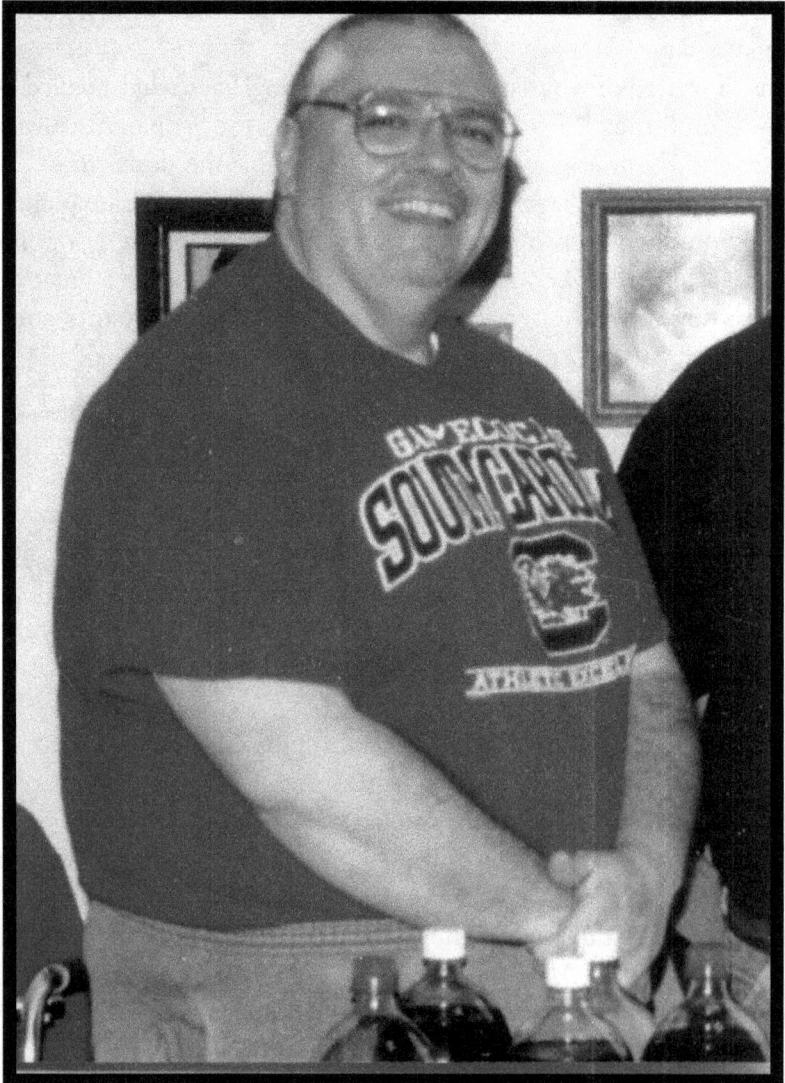

One happy 355-pound soda drinker

PART TWO

◆◇◆◇

MY DIVINE SUPPORT TEAM

There are times when guardian angels are unavailable;
those are the times that God uses special people.

~Anonymous

As you read about the many people and places that formed my divine and essential support system, you may think, "Steve, I do want to change, but I don't know the kind of people you know, and I don't go to the places you go." Don't get discouraged. I've surrounded myself with good people and places. Some of them were prescribed by doctors, like physical therapists, but others I had to choose, like a gym. Surround yourself with the people and places that will help you change. We'll look at how you can identify these people in the next section.

5

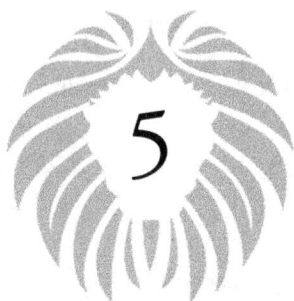

CARING SCIENTISTS

In everyone's life, at some time, our inner fire goes out.
It is then burst into flame by an encounter with another human being.
We should all be thankful for those people
who rekindle the inner spirit.

~Albert Schweitzer

◇◇◇◇

I convinced myself that I was in a hopeless rut. My inner flame had finally gone out and no one had a match big enough to rekindle it. I just gave up and accepted the fact that I would always be obese, even if that meant an early death. There was only one thing I could no longer accept—the excruciating pain in my heel. I really had no choice but to make an appointment with a podiatrist. Apparently, my heel was following in the footsteps of my knees. The burden of supporting 355 pounds severely stressed and inflamed my Achilles tendon, which connects the calf muscle to the heel bone. This tendon is designed to support three-times normal body weight during the strains of daily walking and running. But overuse of this tendon causes Achilles tendonitis, an inflammation that's common among runners and other athletes—but I was just a janitor! In addition to that, X-rays showed the formation of a heel spur, an extra bone that formed under my heel. The bone itself was not painful, but when I walked, it cut into the tissue on the bottom of my foot, and that was excruciating.

My doctor discussed surgery, but first he wanted to try prescribing an expert in the science of healing and the art of caring. Sounds kooky, but that's how the American Physical Therapy Association describes a physical therapist. In August 2007, I limped into the office of TuDor Physical Therapy Centers. There I met my very own caring scientist, Kelly Kovacic. I'd always been tense around medical people, but her energy sparked my spirit and her smile relaxed my nervousness. I felt completely at ease in her presence as we discussed my condition and as I underwent the initial evaluation.

"Do you think losing some weight would help relieve the heel pain?" I asked showing a not-so-firm grasp of the obvious. In the most caring way possible she said, "Dude, are you serious?"

She saw an opening and seized the opportunity. "Perhaps you should try changing your lifestyle."

Whoa, I'd heard that one before. "You don't understand, Kelly," I said. "Over the past thirty years, I've lost more than one hundred pounds three times on three separate diets, and each time I gained back more weight than before."

"That's the problem," she said. "You went on a diet. You need to do something different this time! Every diet you went on succeeded at first but ultimately failed because it only made temporary, external changes (the food you ate) rather than permanent internal changes (how you ate and how you exercised). The amount of weight you lose is not the real goal. Creating a healthy lifestyle is the goal and permanent weight loss is the result. You see, Steve, losing a specific amount of weight will not solve the problems created by your lifestyle, but permanently changing how you eat and exercise will change the quality of your life, and that in turn will solve a lot of your problems."

Kelly could see that my current lifestyle revolved around 24-hour fridge visitations, but she didn't judge me. Instead she offered a solution: "You know, Steve, I've been battling weight loss since the recent birth of my first child, so my husband and I have been seeing a clinical nutritionist to help us both lose weight." She looked me right in the eye and said, "I'll make copies of all the materials we received from the nutritionist and give them to you, but I'm serious here. You have to promise to do the work. You have to want to make a change!"

Oh boy. I could see accountability written all over her, and I could tell that she would follow through with her part of the deal. If I accepted her offer, I knew that I'd be making a commitment to her—the kind of pledge I never before had the courage to make to anyone.

"Okay, Kelly. I'll accept your offer." At least that's what I told her.

"Great, Steve. Just one more thing. I need you to complete this food journal every day and report in each week so we can review it." This was not part of her job, but it was a condition I had to meet if I wanted her help. "It's very important that you write things down. You won't believe how much you eat until you actually write down everything you put in your mouth!" I wasn't looking forward to documenting everything I ate; but I desperately wanted her help, so I sort of did it.

For the first couple of weeks, I showed her bogus journals. I even told her that I lost four pounds in one week, but I really didn't lose anything because I hadn't started the program yet. When I did start, progress was slow. I incorporated only some of the principles and ideas from Kelly's program. As you may have guessed, I had less than stellar results doing things my way, and I felt terrible about lying to the person who was trying to help me change my life. I suppose real change always begins by confronting the real problem—stubbornness, which I had big time.

Part of the program required weighing myself; and like most big people, I hated scales, but Kelly had a plan to deal with that: "It's just too depressing looking at the scale every day, so choose a specific day and only weigh in on that day," she told me. So every Thursday, as soon as I woke up, I went to the bathroom to do my business—that stuff can weigh a lot you know. Then I stepped onto the scale completely naked. Usually, I weighed less in the morning than later in the day.

I highly recommend this strategy for you, too. Why concentrate on daily gains or losses of a quarter pound? Focus, instead, on improving your daily lifestyle long term, just like the contestants who compete on the television program, *The Biggest Loser*. Believe it or not, I had never heard of the show until Kelly mentioned it, "I can't believe you've never seen the show! You have to watch it! It'll be such a boost for you!"

Well, it just so happened that the premiere episode of season four was on that night. I really didn't want to watch it because I don't like reality shows. But I tuned in anyway and just as I'd expected, I didn't like it. Watching big people rumble, bumble, and stumble around on television was not my idea of entertainment. I told Kelly exactly what I thought of the show, but she was adamant: "You've got to give it another shot, Steve. You can't judge it on one episode!" So just for her, I watched episode two and then episode three and was soon addicted.

It's hard to describe just how much that show still means to me even as I write this book. Although I knew many overweight people, none of them were in the process of losing weight by creating a new lifestyle of exercise and balanced eating. Watching real people in real time acknowledge and defeat their obesity consoled and inspired me. It shifted my weight loss efforts into overdrive. In my mind, I was a contestant, too. During my training I experienced every emotion the contestants experienced: anger and happiness, cheers and tears, sadness and gladness. I watched them eat, work out, and get on the dreaded scale each and every week, just like I did. I agonized with them over what the scale would reveal and who would be eliminated. And while the tough and brilliant Jillian and Bob were their coaches, Kelly was mine. It was a team effort now. I did the work. Kelly held me accountable, and *The Biggest Loser* spurred me on. From then on, I fully committed to the weight-loss program and stopped lying to Kelly about it.

I learned a lot from the show, namely that there are no quick fixes and no shortcuts. If I wanted to meet my goals, I had to discipline myself and take Kelly's program seriously. And so I did. I began by eating four to six times a day in smaller portions than usual. I ate a protein and a carb at every meal, such as a boneless, skinless chicken breast and an apple. Three hours later, I ate a can of tuna fish in water and an orange. Three hours later, I had a chef salad with protein and carbs mixed in. I always drank at least four eight-ounce glasses of water with each small meal.

As far as exercise goes, well let's face facts. Working out by yourself can be lonely and difficult. It's tough not having someone right there cheering for you.. The contestants have strict coaches, Jillian and Bob, who support them, care for them, yell at them, and root them on. At physical therapy, Kelly was my Jillian. She didn't yell because she wasn't my trainer and that wasn't her job. She just hovered. For me, that was enough. Try to find a coach or at least a workout partner to hover, yell, or whatever it takes to keep you moving.

After four months of physical therapy and light exercise, such as walking and baby pushups, I had lost sixty-five pounds. I was getting used to a new lifestyle and seeing real results because of it, but good things never last. My physical therapy sessions were about to end, and all I could think about was how I was going to continue losing weight without Kelly. I needed her spark of enthusiasm as much as I needed her to keep me accountable. Fortunately, Kelly's responsibility didn't end when the checks stopped. "You can still come in, tell me about your progress, and work out," she said. "In fact, I really feel you need to do that to sustain your progress."

I couldn't believe anyone would do that for me. Just six months earlier, I had reconciled myself to being fat forever, becoming a cripple, dying an early death, never playing golf again, and believing that would never change. One week later, I met Kelly who, beyond the call of duty, was helping me change all of that. I truly believe she was the work of divine providence—God's guiding hand over one of His lost and defeated creations. I left TuDor that day thinking to myself, *That's the kind of mentor I want to be someday.*

If meeting Kelly weren't providential enough, guess what opened up right next door to TuDor about the same time my physical therapy sessions were ending? A fitness center, otherwise known as *the dreaded gym.* Kelly pointed out that joining a gym would offer me many more exercise options than the limited equipment at TuDor. She even said I could stop in anytime to shoot the breeze with the staff and clients at TuDor who had become my friends. That seriously motivated me because at the time, there was no way I could ever envision myself joining a gym. I imagined kids saying, "Look at the big fat man walking on the treadmill, Mommy," or "This place is really going downhill when they let big guys like that join!" As a custodian, I didn't have a lot of cash lying around to pay for that kind of humiliation. But you know what those thoughts are, don't you? Yeah, that's right, *excuses.* We big people have a million of them.

I was just looking for a way out, but perseverance and self-discipline won. I saved money and just six months after starting physical therapy, I made a long-term commitment by joining my first gym. What a powerful word, *commitment.* It wasn't a secret commitment either. I let everyone know about my gym membership, so I'd have to follow through or else be branded a quitter. I don't commit to a lot of things; but when I do, I don't quit.

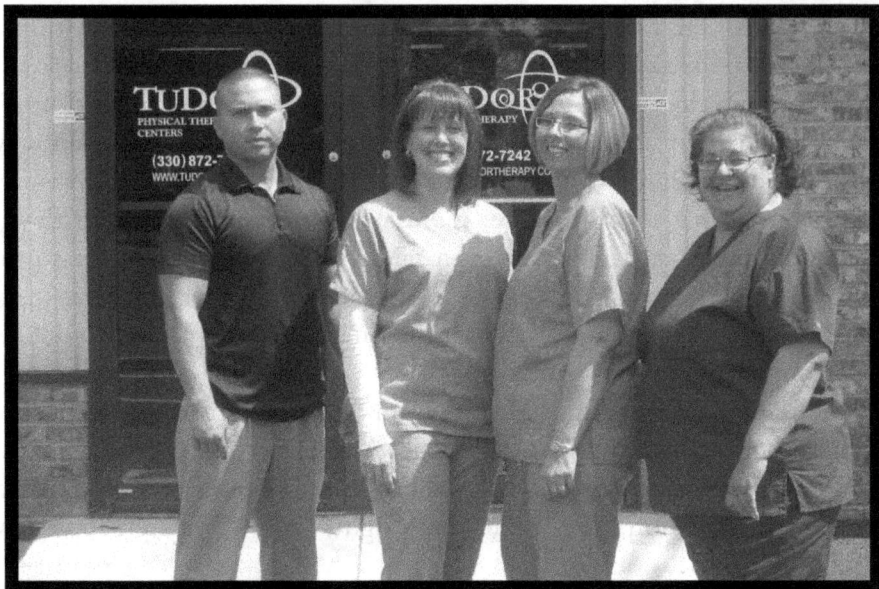

The artful Tudor scientists at Newton Falls, Ohio:
Dan Sharfal, Kelly Kovacic , D.J. Nutt, and Tina Amorganos

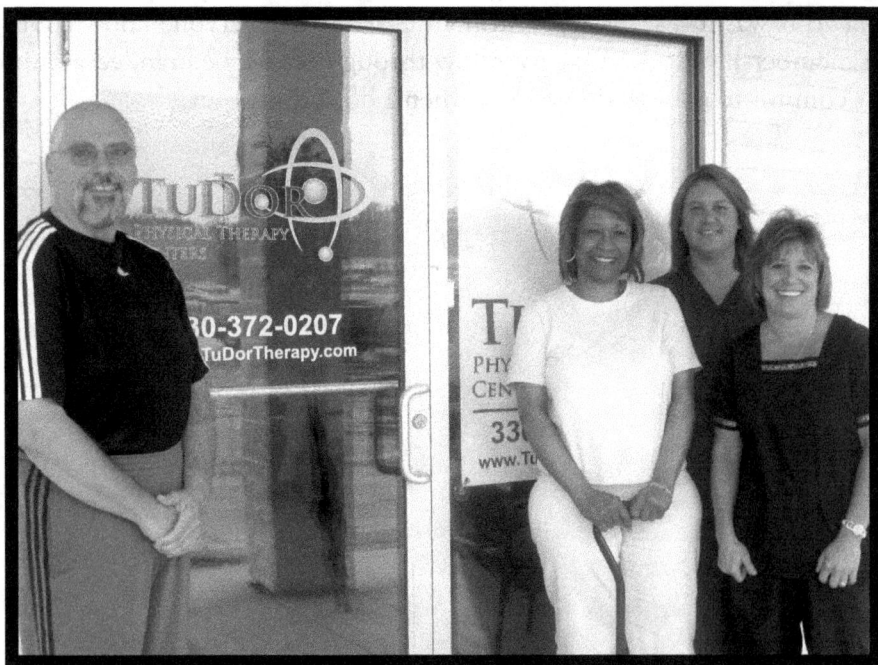

The Warren, Ohio Tudor clan:
Me, Joyce Ringold, Julie Rhodes, and Jeanine Spangler

6

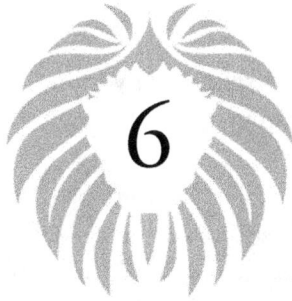

THE DREADED GYM
MY HOME AWAY FROM HOME

*The achievement of your goal is assured the moment
that you commit yourself to it.*
~ *Mack R. Douglas*

I had spent far too many late nights eating like a hog at a trough and getting up the next morning feeling horrible, just like a drunk with a hangover. I had wasted too much time just existing. But once I joined Global Health and Fitness, I became a workout fanatic. The weight just poured off, about four to six pounds a week, and I was having a blast.

I soon developed a support system of professional and compassionate people. One such person was the owner, Bill Myers, who is one chiseled dude. I never understood people who care so deeply about health and fitness until I became rather chiseled myself, relatively speaking, of course. I understand now that gym owners meet a need in their community. Like physical therapists, they help people improve the quality of their lives. And that's what I want to do.

You might have preconceived ideas about what a gym looks like: wood floors, concrete brick walls, poor lighting, and oppressive smells, but they're not all like that. My gym, and many newer clubs, are state-of-the-art facilities with an impressive collection of cardio and strength training equipment, classes for aerobics, yoga, a tanning salon, and sauna, all brightly lit with carpeted floors, paintings, and lots of seating areas to relax and socialize, but that's not why most people go to a gym. They go there to work out.

You might also believe that gyms hire college kids majoring in physical education to greet and train you. Not so at my gym. Ahlam Buss, a bubbly and highly-skilled representative guided me through my very first workout showing me how to correctly use each machine. After we finished, she squatted down and in a very personable way said, "I'm very proud of you for what you've accomplished so far, and I want you to know that I'm here for you if you ever need any help."

What a great thing to say! She had seen lots of people join the gym, go all out for awhile and then slack off, so she encouraged me and even guaranteed that if I kept up the hard work, I'd reach my weight goal in no time. I didn't want her to think I was a slacker, too, so I signed up for three years. How's that for a commitment? I'm determined to train and tone my body religiously at Global. I'll even run there if I ever overindulge. Thankfully it's only a mile away.

Another important part of my Global support team is Eric Bergman, an expert trainer in fitness and nutrition who says they go hand in hand whether you're trying to lose weight, maintain weight, or bulk up. "The two worst inventions ever created were fad diets and scales," Eric told me. "When you're trying to lose weight concentrate on how your clothes fit, not on what the scales say." He also confirmed what Kelly told me: "Diets create temporary changes. You have to change your lifestyle permanently." Those are the two most important lifestyle lessons I've learned on this journey.

I realize I sound like an advertisement for my gym; but unless you live in Ohio, you might never hear of Global Health and Fitness. My point is that the benefits of joining a good gym go far beyond access to exercise equipment. The right gym provides a support staff that's second only to your own personal commitment to change your life.

Okay, now what about all those nasty stares and comments I thought I'd get? Well, I discovered that very few people pay attention to what you or anyone else is doing. Most are just like you—people trying to find their way to health and fitness. They are too busy concentrating on their own workout to notice yours. Really.

So what are you waiting for? What are your excuses? Most gyms are more than willing to set up a payment plan that meets your needs, so there's no financial excuse not to join. Most gyms are open 24/7 and even have day-care centers, so you can fit a workout into your schedule no matter how busy you are. Get up at 4:00 in the morning or come home at 10:00 at night if you have to. There are no excuses. Believe me. I used every excuse in the book before I finally committed myself to a goal. I reminded myself, "If you do what you always did, you'll get what you always got." I was tired of being miserable and just existing. Once I committed myself to a lifestyle change, I suddenly found the time to achieve it.

Since I joined Global, I haven't looked back. It has become my home away from home and the best investment I ever made. It will be yours, too. I promise.

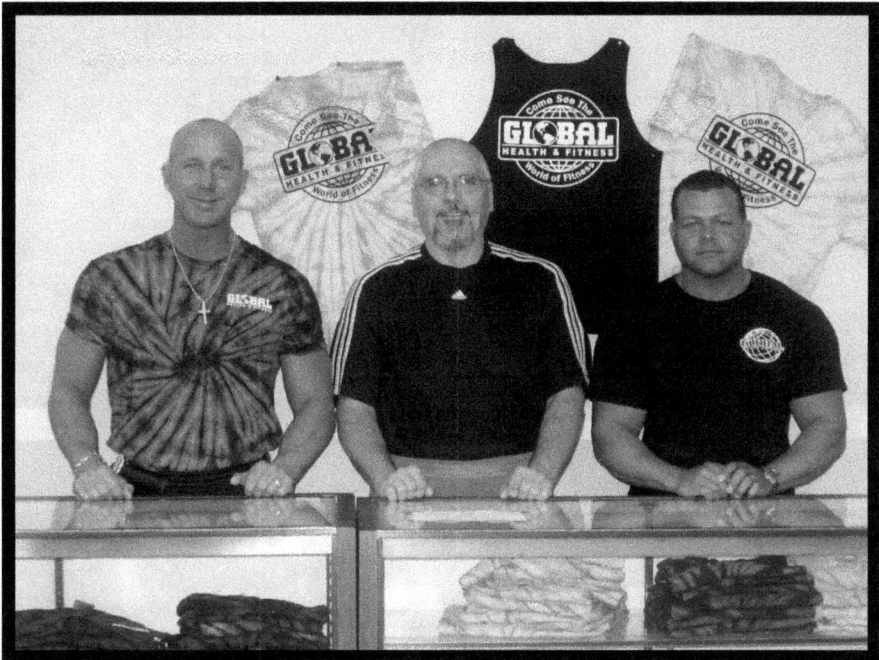

The Global brothers: Bill Myers, Stephen Hosaflook, Eric Bergman

7

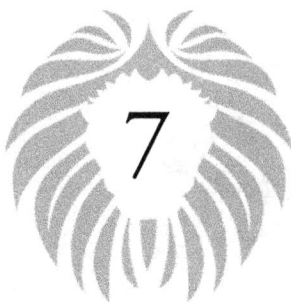

PHYSICAL THERAPY
A PLACE WHERE MIRACLES STILL HAPPEN

*There are only two ways to live your life. One is as though
nothing is a miracle. The other is as though everything is a miracle.*

~Albert Einstein

Physical therapy centers are exceptional places where the talents and skills of physical therapists and their assistants, occupational therapists, and massotherapists produce results that at times are nothing short of miraculous. Maybe you have been prescribed physical therapy or are debating whether it's for you. I can't make that decision for you, but I would like to share how the marvelous work of some inspiring people changed me.

I wasn't sent to TuDor Physical Therapy Center to lose weight because it's not a weight loss clinic. It's a physical therapy center. I just happened to get a kick in the pants while undergoing prescribed therapy. Their motto is "Changing Lives for the Better." Amen to that. I know in my heart I would not be where I am today had it not been for TuDor's tough-but-fair caring scientists, such as Tina Amorganos.

Tina is a little ball of fire with an infectious laugh who did most of the hands-on treatment of my Achilles tendonitis and heel spur. When I say hands on I mean hands on! She knows exactly where to hit the right spot with her massages. "Okay, Steve, take your shoe and sock off, hop up on the table, and lie down on your stomach for me," she would direct me.

It was my very first treatment and so I was a little anxious, but I did whatever she said. Like most first-timers, I remember the exact moment she hit "the spot."

"Aha, I found the magic spot didn't I, Steve?"

"You sure did because that hurt!"

I won't kid you. Every time we had a session together, I knew pain was coming. Tina is a tough taskmaster who doesn't take *no* for an answer, but a sweeter person you couldn't find. It's hard to reconcile the two when you're walking down the hallway and hear the squeals of agony emanating from her dungeon. My curiosity got the better of me during that first week as I stuck my head in her doorway. Tina winked at me and flashed that devilish grin of hers. "Everything's fine, Steve. It's just me, Tina the therapist. It really doesn't hurt that bad. I'm just practicing for my night job, Tina the dominatrix!" That gets laughs every time.

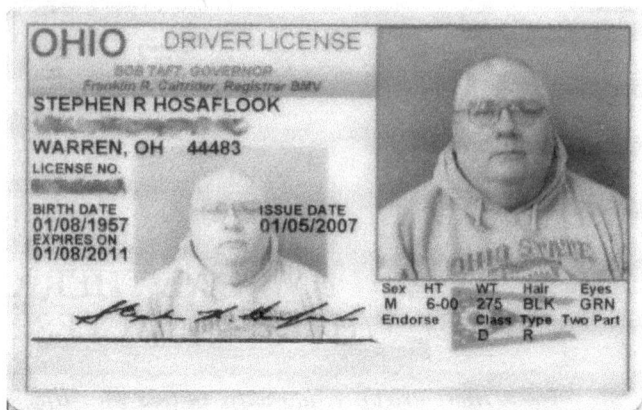

355 pounds

Tina has become one of my biggest cheerleaders, telling new patients about me and what I've accomplished. When I reached 190 pounds, I had to get a new driver's license because I was having trouble proving my identity. To this day, Tina asks me to show before and after licenses to everyone. She gets the biggest kick out of that.

The ladies behind the counter at the Motor Vehicle Department thought it was a big deal, too. They kept looking at the old license and pointing at me. They thought the transformation was so amazing, they even told me I should have been on that show, you know … *The Biggest Loser*.

Getting back to TuDor, Dan Sharfal is one of their massage therapists and a serious body builder. Boy is he chiseled, like one of those professional bodybuilders you see on television. I met him at the end of my treatments when I was still over 300 pounds. He gave me some full body weight exercises to start with and suggestions on how to lift weights, which was so important since I was still a big guy with very little flexibility.

"Let me make this perfectly clear," he said. "You've got to use the correct form when lifting weights! I've been around long enough to see people really injure themselves when they do it wrong!"

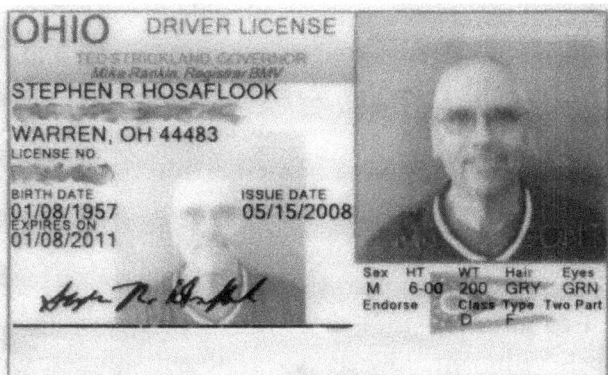

OHIO DRIVER LICENSE

TED STRICKLAND GOVERNOR
Mike Rankin, Registrar BMV

STEPHEN R HOSAFLOOK

WARREN, OH 44483
LICENSE NO

BIRTH DATE   ISSUE DATE
01/08/1957   05/15/2008
EXPIRES ON
01/08/2011

Sex HT   WT   Hair Eyes
M   6-00 200 GRY   GRN
Endorse   Class Type Two Part
           D   F

195 pounds

Less than a month after working out at the gym incorporating his suggestions, I lost thirty pounds.

He would always smile and say, "Looking good, Steve. Keep it up!"

Six months later, just after I hit my goal of 200 pounds, our paths crossed and his jaw hit the floor: "Oh my goodness! Who is this guy? Great job, Steve. You look like a totally different person!"

I can't describe how pumped up I was after that. I love Tina and Dan to death and thank God every day that I had the good fortune to meet them. Imagine that, calling a heel spur and Achilles tendonitis good fortune, but that's the way God works. In fact, I'd gladly go through it again to meet all of the staff at TuDor and clients like the blessed Joyce Ringold.

Joyce always wore a cheerful smile and greeted everyone with a warm hello. She's like my mom in that way. The first time we met, I recall her attractiveness as she sat there, looking rather lifeless in her wheelchair. It was one of those there's something wrong with this picture moments.

In the weeks and months that followed, I saw Joyce gradually progress from the wheelchair, to a walker, and finally to a cane. I thought: *Look at her go. What a driven person she is!* Watching Joyce work so hard made me work even harder. As I slowly learned her story, I became even more inspired; and with her permission, I'll share it here in hopes that you may be inspired, too.

Joyce woke up in the middle of the night feeling nauseated, clammy, and weak, so she headed toward the restroom when her chest tightened as she gasped for air. The next thing she remembered was lying lifeless on the floor. Joyce fell, hit her head on the edge of the bathtub, broke her neck, sustained three fractured cervical vertebrae resulting in spinal cord damage and paralysis. She underwent extensive surgery to remove three discs and insert a metal rod along with some cadaver bones to hold everything together. She spent five weeks in the hospital receiving physical and occupational therapy twice a day.

The doctors told her she would never walk again. At first she cried, then she became angry proclaiming to therapists, doctors, nurses, and anyone else within shouting distance, "I'll show you people. I'm going to walk out of here!"

And so she showed everyone. With the aid of a walker and in front of many who doubted her, she walked out of St. Elizabeth Hospital after five weeks of therapy! There wasn't a dry eye in the house. If that's not a miracle, I don't know what is.

Joyce knew she still had to undergo many months and maybe years of physical therapy. She chose to do so at TuDor—another instance of divine providence. You see, I don't believe in coincidences. God brought all these circumstances and people together in an obvious way so that I would give Him the credit. But wait ... there's more.

Just the other day, I saw Joyce at the gym—my gym. Gosh, did that ever warm my heart. It so uplifted me to see and talk to her. She is a true miracle. The staff at TuDor said that considering what happened to her, Joyce should be dead, but she's very much alive! I watched her ride a stationary bike, walk on the treadmill, and even use a leg press machine. She is determined to throw her cane away and drive her car again.

Through it all, Joyce is still radiant ... and what a smile. Ear to ear. Yet she still can't figure out why people say she inspires them. She doesn't realize how many people have strengthened their self-discipline, grown in personal responsibility, sought accountability, and worked even harder because of her example. I pray every day that God keeps her strong so she can continue her progress. I don't know if she'll ever be 100% functional again; but if not, it won't be for lack of effort.

Joyce is just one of the many success stories at TuDor—and no, not everybody progresses the way she has. Physical therapy is a team effort. The therapist is the coach while the patient is the player. Tina likes to say, "You get out of therapy what you put into it." I know she's right because once I committed to really changing, real change occurred.

Now you know why I still go to TuDor every week. Their vision of "Changing Lives for the Better" has most definitely come true for me. If TuDor Physical Therapy Center is anything like the thousands of therapy centers around the country, then going to physical therapy (if it's medically necessary) will change your life, too.

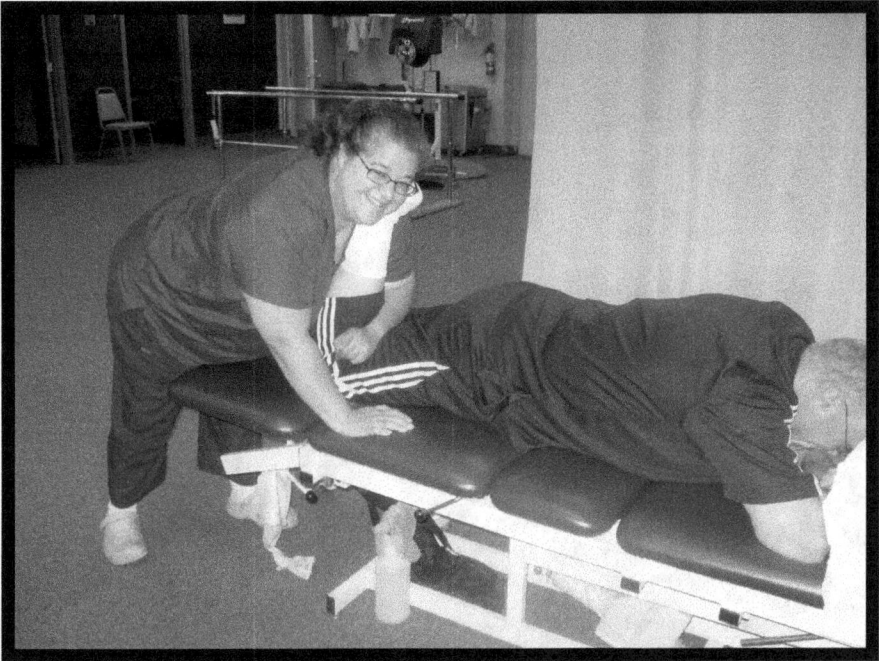

Tina Amorganos working her magical torture

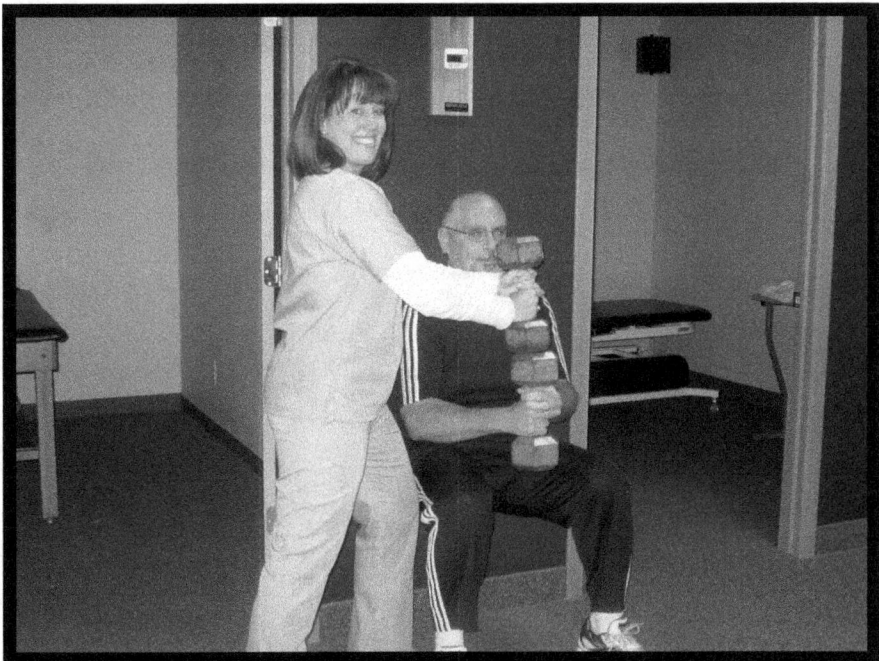

Kelly Kovacic showing her spirit

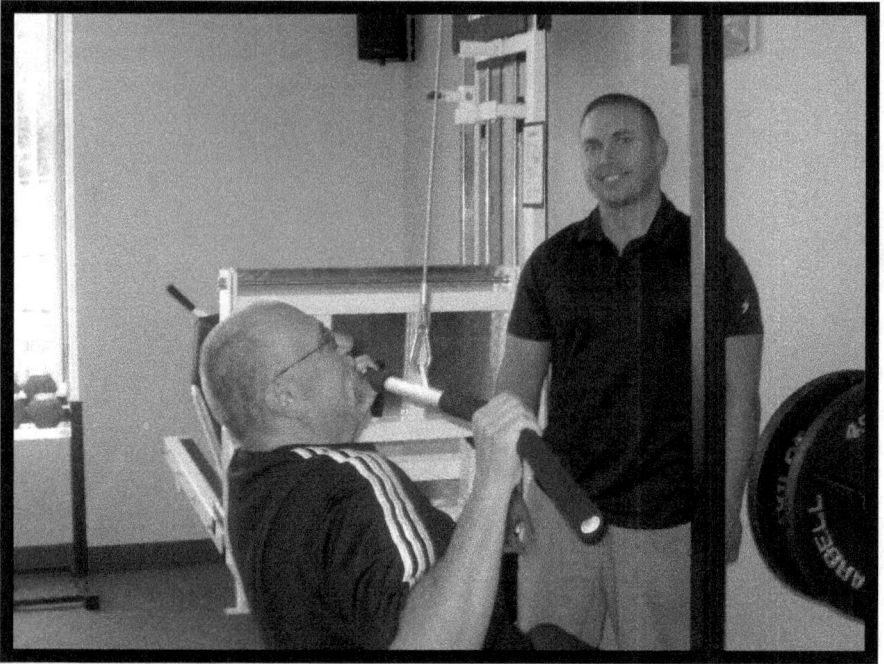

Dan Sharfal trying to make me buff like him

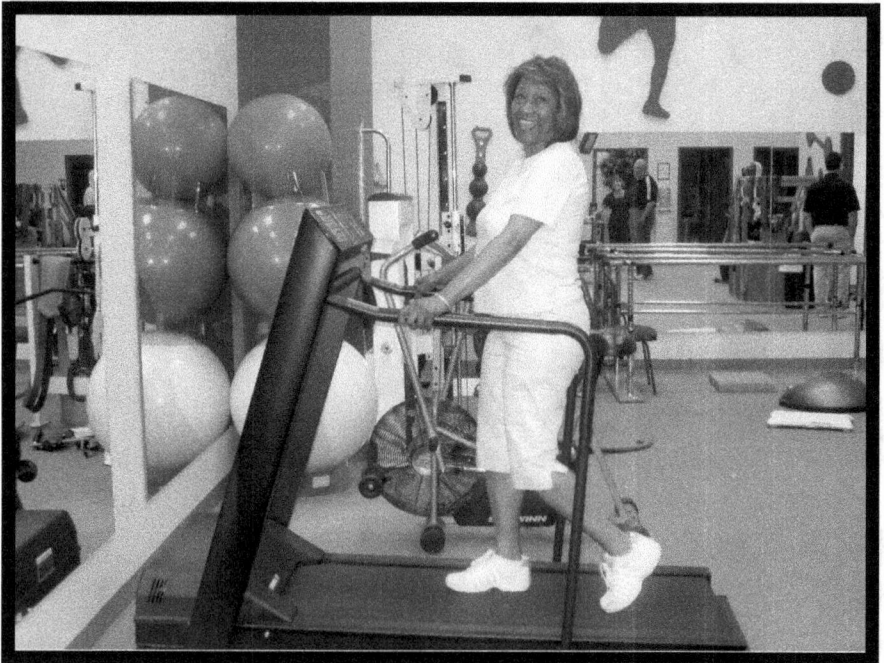

Joyce Ringold proving the doctors wrong

8

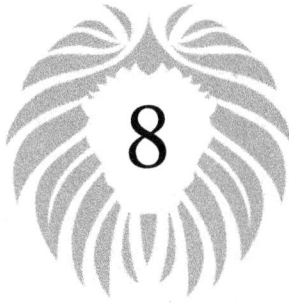

MOM AND DAD
STILL INSPIRING BY EXAMPLE

*You don't really understand human nature unless you know why a child
on a merry-go-round will wave at his parents every time around - and
why his parents will always wave back.*

~ *William D. Tammeus*

◆◇◆◇◆

Some people blame my parents for my obesity, but it wasn't their fault that I became gigantic. While they were in control, they kept me thin. Then I took control, as teenagers do, and became fat. I fell into the same sugar trap that many kids fall into today. I see it every day in the middle school where I work. The kitchen is a business and businesses know how to make money. Sugar makes money, so it's no wonder the popular ala-cart menu has nothing but junk food on it.

As a kid, if I were given the choice between a tuna fish sandwich and a giant chocolate chip cookie, I would have gone for that cookie. And I did, too! As adults, we have a difficult time choosing between tuna and chocolate, so have empathy for your child who has far less self-discipline than you do. Don't leave it up to the school to make sure your child eats a decent, balanced meal. You as the parent must help your children learn how to make right choices for themselves. Here are a few suggestions on how to do that:

- From the day you bring your baby home from the hospital, don't feed him junk food. You wouldn't let him inhale cigarette smoke or drink alcohol, would you?

- In the same way you teach your child how to cross the street safely, also explain the dangers of sugar to their weight, to their teeth, to their complexions, and to their brains. Lovingly help them make wise eating choices wherever they go: at the store, at the restaurant, and at home.

- Train them to exercise self-discipline and temperance in the face of temptation. Help them to choose correctly now so that their risk of diabetes and obesity later is reduced,

- To limit the temptation of junk food, choose a school with a healthy lunch menu and no candy or soda machines.

- Set a good example by making self-disciplined, family-meal choices.

Mom always set a good example by packing our school lunches with balanced meals. At breakfast and dinner, I had to finish everything on my plate or regret it. I stayed thin, though, because the meals were wholesome and only totaled about 1,000-1,500 calories each. Soda, ice cream, chips, and other junk food were treats saved for Friday night and Saturday. I was an active child during this time, so burning those extra calories was a piece of cake.

But I wasn't prepared to handle the freedoms that abound in a middle-school cafeteria. Chocolate milk, sodas, donuts, and whatever the kitchen placed on special became my staple lunch. As I grew (softer and bigger), I spent less time at home and more time enjoying the liberties of eating junk food any time of the day, any day of the week. If I didn't have the cash to buy it, my friends did. One friend regularly collected money from his paper-route customers to buy us all the candy we could handle. Much like teenagers today, we used our intelligence to deceive our parents who had no idea what we were eating. Does that sound like the good ole days for you, too?

Finally, after decades of defiance and arrogance, I am forever changed by the examples my parents continue to set for me every day.

The Toughest Woman I Know

My mom is the absolute toughest woman I know. It's hard to be otherwise when you grow up in the coal towns of West Virginia. Before Mom turned ten, my grandmother, who cooked for miners and loggers, died from cancer. Then my grandfather passed away from a stroke, so my mom's brother and sister-in-law raised her. Her whole purpose and joy in life was raising me and my three siblings. In fact, she didn't work outside the home until my youngest sister entered high school, and she only did so to provide the material things we didn't have growing up. She gave all of her time, talents, and money to her family.

I remember when she hand-sewed bridesmaid gowns for my two sisters' weddings. She even cooked for the receptions and somehow fit in attending the ceremonies, too. She gave, gave, and gave. The way I look at it now, I'm just returning the favor by giving back.

Now weighing in at eighty-five pounds wringing wet, my mom lives with pain 24/7. For thirty-five years, rheumatoid arthritis has been slowly destroying her joints. After fourteen surgeries, which have done little to ease the pain, people ask why she smiles so much. Sometimes I'm not sure; but when I complain about going to the gym to work out, I just look at her smile as she pushes her walker one slow step at a time across the living room, and I ask God to help me have the kind of peace and joy she has. It's a pure joy that comes from knowing for certain that she'll be spending eternity free of all pain in the presence of God. She knows she's not going to heaven because of all the good things she did for us, but because of her sincere trust in Jesus as her personal Savior. Yes, if anyone has a room prepared in heaven, it's my mom, Ethel Hosaflook.

A Man's Man is He

My dad is an ole, tobacco-chewing hillbilly from West Virginia, but a really well-built one. He could've been one of those fitness models you see today. I mean the man was built! And considering his age and health problems, he's still built! When we were kids; we would hang from each of his arms as he stood in one of those show-off-your-biceps poses.

A man's man is my dad. He wanted to fight in Korea, but his high blood pressure disqualified him. Instead, he settled in Ohio and supported his family, the way all great American men do, by working forty-three years at the same factory. I'm very proud of the way he's fighting diabetes, high blood pressure, and dementia. We all know it's a losing battle; even so, he still tries hard to care for Mom but forgets many things and struggles with the resulting shame. He can't help Mom shower anymore because he doesn't remember how, so I do that now. No matter what his daily challenges are, he's still a commanding figure and my greatest hero. I don't think he'll ever know just how much love and respect I have for him.

If my mom and dad can maintain their dignity and joy throughout their daily pain and challenges, I can maintain my weight loss while I joyfully care for them. There's an old saying: "You'd better give them roses while they can still smell them." I do that for my parents every night before going to bed by telling them, "I love you." And they do the same for me. I'm truly proud to be the son of George and Ethel Hosaflook.

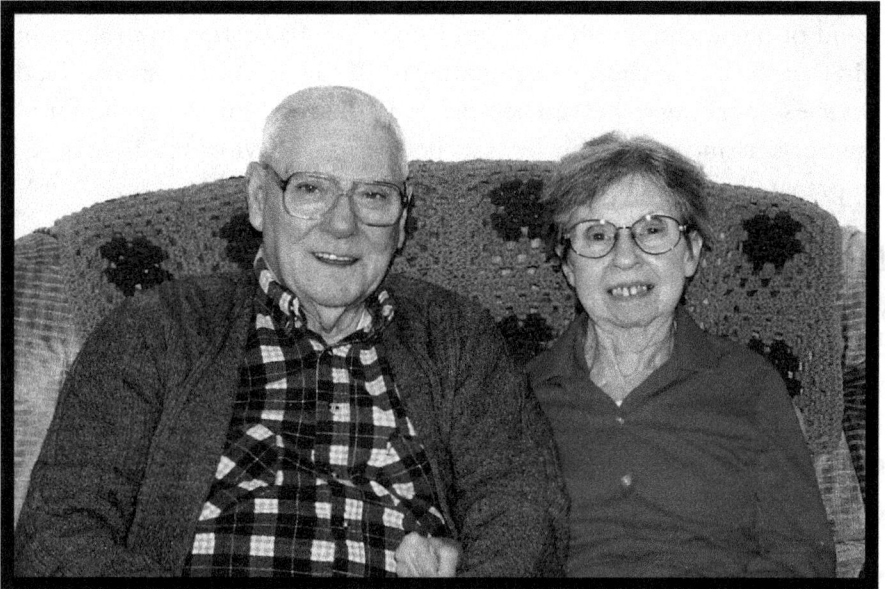

The Inspirational and Joyful George and Ethel Hosaflook

9

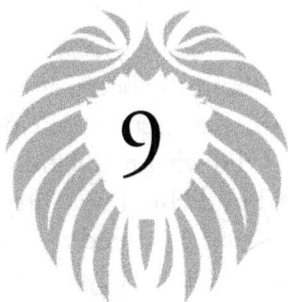

GOD
IN HIM I TRUST

No nation can be strong except in the strength of God,
or safe except in His defense. The trust of our people in God should be
declared on our national coins.

~ Salmon P. Chase, Secretary of the Treasury, 1861

Just as our nation openly declares its reliance on God on the money we carry, I also declare my reliance on God to you because He is the reason I am alive and able to help you through your weight loss journey.

I don't want to preach to you about any one diet or any one religion. I only want to share with you why I believe I am alive and thin again. You see, I believe that every good thing on earth comes from God, like me meeting Kelly and you reading this book. And even though I think I'm a really good person, compared to the perfect God, I really miss the mark in every way. Although I want to help you change your life, that won't get me into eternity with God. What will get me to heaven is my faith that Jesus made me good in His eyes when He died on the cross and paid the price for my sinful nature. His forgiveness of my sins and my obedience to Him grants me entrance to my own room in heaven instead of a swim in the lake of fire. I know that seems like a bunch of hooey to many people, but I believe the Bible is an accurate description of God's plan for my life.

Of course bad things happen, too, like my obesity and my parents' illnesses, but I don't believe that all bad things come from God. My obesity developed because of a lack of self-discipline. If I were truly obedient to God, I would have tried hard to control my gluttony and actively seek to live a more holy life. My parents' illnesses are probably a result of their own lifestyle choices in addition to generations of hereditary issues.

When I think about all the really bad things that should have happened to me, I realize how good God has been in spite of my life-long disobedience. When I was seven years old, I did what many kids in Sunday school do. I asked Jesus to come into my heart. I told Him I was sorry for my sins and then I went on my merry way doing whatever I wanted to do—and you've read how that turned out. Instead of obeying God, I obeyed my belly. In spite of myself, He blessed me beyond anything I was worthy of.

For starters, I should have severe diabetes or heart disease by now considering how horribly I treated my body. I let my own desires control my destiny for so long; but finally, God directed my steps to TuDor and Global. I know it was Him, because only God could coordinate all those circumstances so perfectly. Why now? Why not twenty years ago? Maybe He tried and I rejected His offer because my eyes were closed to His plan. I wanted to do what I wanted to do. But now I see clearly. That's even more miraculous than the weight loss. I'm not only thin again, I also see His purpose for me—I must help people who are obese and whenever possible, help them to give God the glory.

Maybe God has been directing your steps all along. That's what Proverbs sixteen, verse nine says He does; but like me, your eyes and ears were not yet tuned in to His frequency. Perhaps now you are more receptive.

Did you know that if you delight in God's Word and His will, He will give you the desires of your heart? That's what Psalm 37 says and I believe it. So where do you start? Find a Bible-centered church that teaches about the God of the Bible. Ask God to show you His way and not somebody else's way and He will let you find Him.

PART THREE

◆◇◆◇◆

TAKE ACTION

We can't become what we need by remaining what we are.
~ Max Dupree

10

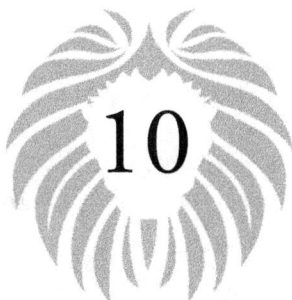

PUTTING AMERICAN VALUES TO WORK

Americanism means the virtues of courage, honor, justice, truth, sincerity,
and hardihood—the virtues that made America.

~ Theodore Roosevelt

◈◈◈◈

Losing 160 pounds and keeping it off would not be possible without a support team and belief in good old-fashioned American values. Now it's time to put people and values to work for you. Allow me to ask you some hard questions— important questions that will help you lay a solid foundation for true change. We are going to answer them together, me as a 355-pound janitor just a year ago and you today. Use the space provided for your answers or answer on a separate sheet of paper, but do answer them. Here we go . . .

Acknowledge the Truth

You've seen yourself in the mirror. You know how much you weigh. You're even reading a book about losing 160 pounds in a year, but do you really believe you're morbidly overweight? Do you really believe all those bad things that doctors say will happen to you? Do you know why you live in pain?

How much do you weigh?

Me: 355 pounds   You:_____

On the left column, list the physical ailments you have, which are probably due to being overweight. On the right column, list the physical ailments that doctors say you will get if you don't lose weight.

Me: Severe osteoarthritis, Early death   You: _____

45

Pursue Liberty

Liberty is to the collective body, what health is to every individual body. Without health no pleasure can be tasted by man; without liberty, no happiness can be enjoyed by society. ~ Thomas Jefferson

As Americans, we each have a right to pursue life, liberty, and happiness, like bending down to tie your shoes without losing your breath, walking up stairs pain free, or playing a full round of golf in the heat. I am so thankful to live in a country where I can be happy and free to enjoy the perks of daily slimness. One day you will be, too.

What is your ideal weight?

Me: 190 pounds _____   You: _____

List activities that you would like to perform but can't because of your physical ailments and weight.

Me: Walk up the stairs pain-free.   Sit in one seat. _____

You: _____

Accept Responsibility for Your Obesity

You must take personal responsibility. You cannot change the circumstances, the seasons, or the wind, but you can change yourself. That is something you have charge of. ~Jim Rohn

You must assign the blame for your obesity to the true cause of your obesity. Until you take responsibility for being overweight, you will never take responsibility for losing weight.

Okay, this might be tough. List the reasons and excuses you made this week for eating that carton of ice cream, that double-double cheeseburger, that three-cheese pizza … and everything else.

Me: Lost game of golf.   Won game of golf. _____

You: _____

Seek Accountability and Support

Too often we underestimate the power of a touch, a smile, a kind word, a listening ear, an honest compliment, or the smallest act of caring, all of which have the potential to turn a life around. People come into our lives for a reason, a season, or a lifetime. Embrace all equally. ~ Leo Buscaglia

Losing 100 pounds completely on your own efforts is definitely doable. I did it three times, but I would not have changed my lifestyle without a divine support team. Now you might say, "I don't believe in God," or you might say, "God didn't give me a Kelly to kick my butt or a Tina to show me off to people." Maybe He has or maybe He will and you just don't know it yet.

You don't have to wait around for someone to knock on your door or for God to give you a vision. There are people who would love to save your life from earthly destruction—to be your Kelly, if only you would ask. Wouldn't you want to be a mentor to someone you care about? Is there a teacher, neighbor, friend, or relative who will keep you on track? Is there someone you admire so much that you will not let them down?

List the people you would like to report to during your lifestyle change:

Me: <u>Kelly at TuDor.   Global Fitness trainers.</u>

You: _____

Choose one or two of these special people and ask them something like this: "I really want to lose weight for good, but I'm not sure I can do it completely on my own. Would you hold me accountable to following a new plan of eating and exercising? I really want to permanently change my lifestyle, but I need your help and support for the first several months." Then explain the program to them. Make sure they know your exercise and nutrition plan. Educate them about your program so they can honestly make you accountable. For example, make a regular appointment every week to show them your journal. Without this accountability, you might let several days go by without writing anything in it.

Everyone needs a personal cheerleader. Joining support groups online, such as SparkPeople.com and TheFatBurnFiles.com. or in person at hospitals and weight loss clinics are incredibly helpful, but be careful of the type of group you join. I will not join a group unless they put the blame squarely where it belongs—on me. It's my fault that I became obese, and it will be my fault if it happens again. Your support group must recognize that and hold you accountable for it.

Be Courageous

God grant me the serenity to accept the things I cannot change; courage to change the things I can; and wisdom to know the difference.

~ *Serenity Prayer*

I used to be one of the least courageous people you could ever meet. I had courage to commit to friends, to a job, to caretaking for my parents, but I had no courage to overcome fears, to better my education or job, to lose weight for good, to change the things I could change. Then I saw others overcome far worse disabilities than obesity, like Nick Vujicic, a valiant man born without arms and legs. He dedicates his life to changing what he can change, joyfully and fearlessly. Infuse yourself with his courage by watching Nick do what he does best at LifeWithoutLimbs.org.

Gain hands-on courage by volunteering at a rehabilitation center or nursing home. There you'll see amputees, the paralyzed, and the elderly learning how to walk again through sheer will, perseverance, and faith. They're also changing what they can.

I have changed what I could change: The food I eat. The exercise I perform. The weight I lost. These accomplishments gave me the courage to conquer a life-long fear of falling from great heights. In one weekend, I not only took my first plane ride, I also rode the Albuquerque Sandia Peak Tramway, a 2.7 mile trip up to 10,000 feet. For me, that's double courage!

What fears or life situations would you like to overcome?

Me: <u>Heights.   Writing a book.</u>_____

You: _____

Who do you admire for their courage and why?

_____

_____

Persevere for a Purpose

Persevere: to persist in a state, enterprise, or undertaking in spite of counter-influences, opposition, or discouragement. ~ *Merriam-Webster.com*

"Perseverance" is such a powerful word. You might want to quit many times, but you're not going to. Instead, you will remember all the things you can't do because of your obesity. You'll remember the arthritis, the tendonitis, the diabetes, and the heart conditions you have now or will have later because of the way you neglected your body for decades.

No matter how difficult the workouts become, you will remember how difficult it is to be fat, to be denied the simple pleasures of life because you are "handicapped"—another great word. It means you have a disadvantage that makes success more difficult. That's right. Your obesity is a great disadvantage. You probably don't go to the county fair, or take a trip to Europe, or even play miniature golf because it's too painful to walk, to climb stairs, or to stand in the heat. You can't really play with your kids like they want you to, sit comfortably in an airplane seat, or even tie your shoes. You get the picture.

The contestants on *The Biggest Loser* persevere because of coaches like Jillian and Bob. When the contestants go back to the rigors of work and home life, they continue competing with the support of spouses or friends, not to mention a $250,000 grand prize to the biggest loser. I'd probably persevere for $250,000 and you probably would, too, but we don't have that kind of motivation to keep us going. Ultimately, we have to persevere for a greater purpose.

My purpose:

As a Christian, I must care for my body, grow in self-discipline, and obey His will for my life. My body is His temple, so for Him, I will stay fit and trim forever.

What is your purpose? What is the one reason above all other reasons that you want to become fit and trim forever?

_____

_____

_____

_____

_____

Be Self-Disciplined

How do you go from where you are to where you want to be? I think you have to have an enthusiasm for life. You have to have a dream, a goal, and you have to be willing to work for it. Don't give up, don't ever give up!
~ Jim Valvano

Jim Valvano became famous for coaching college basketball for nineteen years. Then one day a doctor told him he had a year to live. In that last year, he never lost his enthusiasm or self-discipline regardless of his deteriorating health. He became a mentor to thousands of cancer patients encouraging them to persevere as well as building public awareness of the condition. He motivated himself by saying, "I'm not giving up! It's going to be hard every day, but I'm not giving up!" If a man with a year to live can say that and mean it, so can you! No day will be perfect, but regardless of the mistakes you make, strive for excellence.

I also love what Ralph Waldo Emerson said, "Finish each day and be done with it ... you have done what you could, some blunders and absurdities have no doubt crept in; forget them as soon as you can. Tomorrow is a new day; you shall begin it well and serenely."

For me, perseverance comes down to mind over matter. *I will go to the gym! I will eat wisely today! I will help someone else today that will take my focus off of me!* I have to say these things to myself every day and I will, no doubt, have to say them every day for the rest of my life, especially when my emotions say: *it's okay to eat a half-gallon of mint chocolate chip ice cream and drink a liter of root beer while watching TV tonight. Go ahead and stop at that market. You deserve a break today.*

I've shared the quotes that motivate me to persevere. What quote or Bible verse motivates you to stay focused on your goals in difficult and challenging times?

_____

_____

Work Hard

Do not wait; the time will never be "just right." Start where you stand, and work with whatever tools you may have at your command, and better tools will be found as you go along. ~ *Napoleon Hill*

You might think that hard work starts at the gym. No. It starts with incorporating the values of truth, personal responsibility, accountability, courage, perseverance, and self-discipline. Remember, physical exercise releases endorphins that create a natural high. You're going to love that, but creating new habits in thought and action is hard. The older you get, the harder it is. I'm fifty-one years old and I did it. I know you can, too.

Guess what? That work starts right now.

11

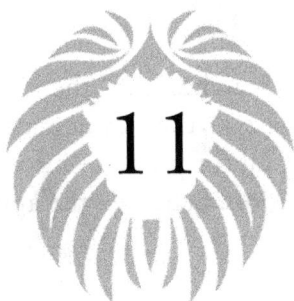

START RIGHT NOW

The secret of getting ahead is getting started. The secret of getting started is breaking your complex overwhelming tasks into small manageable tasks, and then starting on the first one.

~ Mark Twain

◇◆◆◇

Now that you've prepared yourself for what lies ahead and have committed to work to change your lifestyle, the time to start is now.

Develop a Program

How do you develop a lifestyle change program? You might devise one on your own based on personal research in libraries or on the Internet. That's fine as long as you don't think up another quick-fix, starve-your-body-of-vital-nutrients kind of program. You need to inform yourself about how food and exercise impacts your life. As you start the journey, seriously consider hiring a dietician, fitness trainer, or wellness center to tailor a program just for you and to monitor your progress. Ask people you respect for referrals, such as your doctor, friends, and colleagues who have successfully followed a program of life-style change.

Finding a program is not difficult. Overcoming the mental block that keeps you from finding a program is often debilitating, so let's begin now. Write down the names of people who have successfully followed weight-loss programs and could give you a reliable referral.

_____

_____

_____

From referrals, Internet searches, and the phone book, write down the names of three people who are in the business of designing and monitoring life-style change programs. Call for program information and pricing. Set up an appointment for consultation. Schedule the appointment in your planner. And go to the appointment.

Name of person or business: _____

Phone Number: _____

Appointment date and time: _____

Notes: _____

_____

Name of person or business: _____

Phone Number: _____

Appointment date and time: _____

Notes: _____

_____

Make a decision. Which program will you choose?

_____

_____

When will you start?

_____

_____

Who will be your accountability partner?

_____

_____

Manage Your Time

Because I work as a full-time custodian for a public middle school and am the primary caregiver for two elderly parents with debilitating illnesses, I do the laundry, the cooking, the bathing, the shopping, and any other chore you can think of for my parents and for myself. On top of all of that, I work out at the gym and cook healthy meals for the week. How do I find this time? By getting rid of unhealthy, time-wasting tasks, like eating all the time at restaurants, at home, and at stores.

Below is a typical weekday schedule before my lifestyle change:

Before My Lifestyle Change	
Time	**Task**
8:00 a.m.	Get up. Go to McDonalds for Two Egg McMuffins, two hash browns, a cinnamon roll, and breakfast soda.
9:00 a.m.	Home chores
10:00 a.m.	Eat bowl of sweet cereal and two toasted cheese sandwiches. Wash that down with a couple of cans of Coke
11:00 a.m.	Errands
12:00 p.m.	Stop at Wendy's on my way to work to get a double hamburger with cheese, large fries, and a large root beer.
1:00 – 10:00 p.m.	My co-worker and I typically share an extra large pizza for lunch. She eats two pieces and I eat the rest. During the evening at work, I visit the kitchen several times to munch on cookies, cakes, pies, chips, basically anything I could find.
10:00 p.m.	Stop at the store on the way home from work to buy ice cream, potato chips, and a soda,
11:00 p.m.	Watch TV while eating ice cream, potato chips and soda.
1:00 a.m.	Go to bed

The next page shows a revised weekday schedule after my lifestyle change.

After My Lifestyle Change	
Time	**Task**
8:00 a.m.	Wake up and make breakfast for my parents. Have two slices of toasted rye bread with a tablespoon of unsalted chunky peanut butter. I drink a protein powder shake that I mix in a blender with a heaping teaspoon of my favorite amino acid powder, nonfat milk or water, and sometimes a favorite fruit.
8:30 a.m.	At the gym, on a heavy weight-training day, I'll go through my upper body workout. I follow that with a twenty-two minute session of interval cardio training.
10:00 a.m.	At home, I heat up a boneless six-ounce pork loin chop on two slices of whole grain, whole wheat bread.
11:00 a.m.	Doctor appointments
12:00 p.m.	Run errands
1:00 p.m.	At home, I eat a fourteen-ounce chef salad from the local supermarket and then it's off to work.
2:00 p.m.	Home chores
3:00 p.m.	At work I'll have two more meals three hours apart. First up, I'll have a four-ounce boneless skinless chicken breast with a side salad.
6:00 p.m.	At work, my second meal might be another chicken breast with a piece of fruit. I mix it up every day, but every meal contains a protein and a carb.
10:15 p.m.	At the gym after work, I'll do a 22-minute session of interval cardio training on the recumbent stationary bike.
11:00 p.m.	At home, I take care of Mom and get her to bed. Watch some TV.
midnight	Go to bed.

You may have never thought about everything you do every day and how much time it takes out of your day, such as going to the store to buy junk food, going to the restaurant to eat junk food, preparing unhealthy meals, eating unhealthy meals, watching TV, talking on the phone, playing games, or searching the Internet. You just know that you have no time to exercise, but you will find time if you keep a calendar to schedule all of your daily tasks, including exercise and eating. Take a moment now to complete a typical weekday schedule for your life today and what it can be after your lifestyle change:

Before Your Lifestyle Change

Time	Task
7:00 a.m.	
8:00 a.m.	
9:00 a.m.	
10:00 a.m.	
11:00 a.m.	
12:00 p.m.	
1:00 p.m.	
2:00 p.m.	
3:00 p.m.	
4:00 p.m.	
5:00 p.m.	
6:00 p.m.	
7:00 p.m.	
8:00 p.m.	
9:00 p.m.	
10:00 p.m.	

After Your Lifestyle Change

Time	Task
7:00 a.m.	
8:00 a.m.	
9:00 a.m.	
10:00 a.m.	
11:00 a.m.	
12:00 p.m.	
1:00 p.m.	
2:00 p.m.	
3:00 p.m.	

4:00 p.m.	
5:00 p.m.	
6:00 p.m.	
7:00 p.m.	
8:00 p.m.	
9:00 p.m.	
10:00 p.m.	

Keep a Journal

Refining my schedule in this way took months and only after a fair amount of kicking and screaming on my part did my day run like a well-oiled machine. I started by keeping track of everything I ate and the exercises I completed each day. At first I journaled lies; and at first, I had few results. Honest journaling killed the deception that I relied on for so long and gave birth to serious weight loss. Whenever I gain weight today, you can bet I have also stopped journaling. When I start journaling again, the weight loss resumes. It takes me about fifteen minutes a day to keep the journal current, and it's not easy. It's one more new habit to form, but it is a critical part of my success.

There's no one right way to keep this journal. You can use a preprinted form like the one in Appendix D or make up your own in a regular notebook. The only requirement is that you truthfully write down exactly what you eat and what exercises you perform. The program you choose will dictate what you eat and how you exercise. Every program, though, starts with the first step.

Take the First Step

When I weighed 355 pounds, it was all I could do just to walk. Because of the excruciating pain in my knees from bone rubbing against bone and in my foot from walking on a protruding heel spur with inflamed tendons, each step evolved into a miserable limp. And as much as I agonized over the idea, I knew I had to get up and start moving. That old saying is true: *Use it or lose it.* Well, I had lost it all.

I forced myself to start walking. I know some who walk at the mall or around their work complex, but I started at a nearby park and later at the athletic track of a local school. I set my initial walking goal at an hour a day and

I met that goal by slowly walking two thirty-minute sessions. It didn't matter how far I walked. My goal was to walk one hour every day, and I did.

Around that time, Kelly and Tina recommended calf stretches and other exercises to strengthen the Achilles tendon and guess what happened? The more I strengthened the area around the Achilles tendon, the faster I walked. The more I walked, the more the pounds came off. As the pounds came off, the walking became easier. I gradually worked my way up from a one-mile crawl to a brisk, non-stop three-mile trek every day!

Where can you walk safely for one hour a day?

_____

_____

_____

Would you like a walking partner? Who can you ask?

_____

_____

_____

Work Out at Home

Walking is still one of my favorite exercises, but once I conquered that workout challenge, I moved on to full-body exercises: pushups, wall squats, and planks. At first I couldn't do the flat-on-the-floor pushup, so I used the stairs at home and at work. Whenever I had five minutes to spare, I'd do ten incline pushups (which was so much easier than flat on the floor pushups). The stronger I got, the more pushups I could complete until I finally graduated to the Marine pushup. Anytime I had a break at home or at work, I'd drop and do ten to fifteen pushups ten to twenty times a day.

I also did the plank, which is similar to a pushup but is actually an abdominal exercise. Lying on my elbows, I push myself up so the only body parts touching the floor are my elbows and toes. At 355 pounds, I could only hold that position for thirty seconds and even that was very tough. At 190 pounds and physically fit, I can now hold myself up for five minutes! How about that?

If you are not a Marine-kind of exerciser, that's okay. Don't forget about all those exercises you did in Phys. Ed. class, like sit-ups, jumping jacks, and deep knee bends. They still work and are available to you anytime, anywhere for free.

If I had to recommend only one piece of equipment to buy, it would be the versatile and always entertaining stability ball. I use it every day and believe me, it's the best twenty bucks I ever spent. You can do just about any exercise with this ball. I do 150 crunches on it twice a day as well as push-ups, planks, and wall squats, too. Sometimes I sit on it while writing this book because balancing myself on it strengthens my abdominal muscle and lower back. That means when I forget what I'm sitting on and don't use my abs correctly, I roll right off! So be patient while you learn how to use it properly. Each ball comes with an instruction DVD and workout plan, but first make sure to buy a ball that's the right size for you, which is determined by your height. Check your local sporting goods store. I bought mine at Walmart.

What exercises can you do for free or for minimal cost at home?

_____

_____

Join a Gym

Once I conquered these basic full-body-weight exercises, I graduated to working out on the equipment at the physical therapy center and then at the gym: stationary bikes, the treadmill, and a Nautilus machine for weight resistance training, such as biceps curls and triceps pull downs. You'll need to join a gym to use machines like these. There's no way around it.

Maybe you can't afford the monthly or annual fee of a gym, and I understand that completely. Remember, I'm a custodian and not rich by any stretch of the imagination; but my health was too important not to take this most important step in my weight-loss program, so I saved up and joined. Most clubs have several membership options with a wide range of prices, so shop around until you find one you can afford. Besides, what price do you put on your health?

I know that most communities have many fitness centers to choose from, so here are some tips for finding your own home away from home:

- Ask for a tour of the facility and take note of how caring and compassionate the staff is. If you feel the staff is giving you a sales job and not a personal invitation to change your life, look elsewhere.

- Look for staff who work out and help clients work out.

- Look for a popular gym. If no one is working out there, others probably know something you don't.

- Are most of the clientele working out or socializing? A gym is a social place for some people. You can't avoid that. But don't allow the people in the gym to distract you from actually working out.

- Walk up to people who are not working out and ask them what they like and dislike about the gym.

- Walk around every area of the facility. Is it clean? Look for a gym with a regular cleaning crew rather than staff who clean whenever they have a moment.

Joining a gym was exactly what I needed when I needed it because it gave me the opportunity to increase the variety and intensity of my workouts. At first, though, I didn't know what the heck I was doing, so I truly appreciated all the help and training everyone gave me. Let's face it. Everyone at a gym is fighting the same physical fitness battle and most people are happy to help if you ask. And I asked often.

If you truly can't afford a membership right now, continue walking and exercising at home until you are able to save enough money to join.

Plan Your Workout

Every day before I leave for the gym, I journal exactly what machines I'm going to use, how much weight I'll start out with, and how many sets I'm going to do. You won't know how to do this yet, but you will learn by experimenting, by asking trainers, and watching chiseled dudes. My own exercise regimen is described in Appendix B.

Be Patient during the Plateaus

I lost four to six pounds a week when I started working out at the gym, and I really was having a blast. Then for two straight weeks, I only lost one lousy pound a week! I moped around TuDor for several days as I reluctantly stretched and exercised. Of course, Kelly noticed and said, "You look like someone who just lost his best friend. What's the problem?"

So I told her about my despair. Keep in mind that I was at a physical therapy center and over the four months there, I had come to know many of the clients undergoing therapy for strokes, heart attacks, joint replacement surgeries, and more serious problems. And there I was, whining about only losing two pounds.

Kelly has a knack for not candy-coating things and announced to the entire clientele, "Okay everybody. Let's all have a pity party for Steve. He only lost two pounds in the last two weeks. Poor guy! He only *lost* two pounds!" Then she looked right at me and said, "Steve, don't you get it? You *lost* two pounds! You didn't stay the same and you didn't gain. You *lost* two pounds!"

Well, I was pretty embarrassed, so I apologized to everyone immediately. I learned a valuable lesson that day. Don't be a whiner! Some patients in that center looked to me for motivation, and I let them down that day. Never again! That's why I continue to go to TuDor every week, to motivate and to be motivated.

Kelly knocked me down that day; but before I left the center, she pulled me aside to offer candid advice to lift me back up. You see, I was depressed because I wasn't losing weight, like the people on *The Biggest Loser* TV show. I'm a competitor at heart and I thought I wasn't winning or even keeping up. She gently explained, "Steve, you don't have access to a physical trainer six hours a day. You are accomplishing great things all on your own while still caring for your parents and working a full-time job."

That was a very special teacher/student moment. She made me see I was actually doing better than the people on the show. To help me get over this temporary setback, Kelly suggested changing some things in my eating regimen, like adding a little more protein and taking away some carbs a few days a week. She also suggested making a change in my workout routine and eating schedule. Sure enough, I got right back on track. Changing things around a little has become a standard course of action in my daily exercise and eating regimen.

Ups and downs register loudly on the scale and in my heart, but there is no way around it. Changing my lifestyle has been a roller-coaster ride. It's painful. It's exhilarating. It's worth every tear shed in pain and joy.

My exercise regimen has come a long way since taking those first slow steps around the track just over a year ago, and yours will come a long way, too, but it will not begin until you take that first step.

Change the Way You Eat

Exercise helped me get out of the mess I made for myself, but it's really only 25% of the battle. Choosing the right food comprises the remaining 75%. Exercise must be a critical part of any program, but it all comes down to what we put in the old pie hole that really makes the difference. If you burn 5,000 calories a day through regular exercise, but keep eating 10,000-20,000 calories a day, not much is going to change except that you'll get bigger. Do you know that when you exercise regularly, you won't want to eat as much junk as you do now? Your body is going to crave healthier food to nourish it. Even so, re-learning how to eat was the toughest part of this whole program for me and it might be for you, too.

First of all, don't drink your calories! I don't drink anything that has calories in it anymore. I only drink water, water, and more water! Almost 70% of your body is composed of water. It is essential for regulating your body's temperature, transporting nutrients throughout the blood stream, removing waste, and preventing dehydration, which can happen fairly easily while working out. It also keeps your body from confusing hunger with thirst, which is very common. Sometimes you eat when you are actually thirsty. Drink water and stop being thirsty.

As for food, I know some of you might be thinking about starving yourself. Please don't do that. Your body needs fuel to power the fat-burning process. It takes fuel to burn fat, but good fuel. Good carbs, not bad carbs. An apple, not a bowl of ice cream. You know the difference between what is good and bad food. You just have to choose it. Try to use food for fuel, not comfort. Believe me, I know it's hard, but in order to change your body size, you have to change your attitude about food. Eat to live. Don't live to eat.

Too many diets create dangerous imbalances in your body because they usually restrict some important ingredient that it needs for fuel. The Atkins diet severely restricts carbohydrates, which is good in some ways and dangerous in others. The human body needs carbohydrates for fuel, especially when you're working out. With this in mind, I recommend any weight-loss program that includes plenty of lean protein, complex carbohydrates such as whole grains, potatoes, beans, green leafy vegetables, fresh fruit, and good fats found in fish and nuts. This is a balanced diet that can be continued forever, not just while you're losing weight.

I started my new way of eating by replacing refined sugar (or anything including refined sugar) with fresh fruit, natural sugars, and good carbs. As time went on, I tried eating new foods—foods I was sure that I'd never eat, like brown rice. I even bought a rice cooker! I can't get enough of it now. And yams! Pop those babies in the microwave for a few minutes then bake them in the oven with some nutmeg and cinnamon. Mmm, mmm, great!

Of course, there will be certain foods you're not fond of. I still can't eat oatmeal. Mom told me I wouldn't even eat it when I was a baby, I'd just spit it out. So I don't eat it, but I do make healthy eating enjoyable and delicious. Most of all, I was amazed at how good food could taste without adding sugar and salt to it. Instead of these weight gaining chemicals, I now add natural spices like cumin, cilantro, and turmeric to my meals, and I love it.

Study cookbooks and web sites about healthy eating, but always keep in mind this one basic truth: if you want to lose weight, you have to create a caloric deficit. That simply means you have to burn more calories than you consume by combining sensible eating habits with exercise. There's just no way around it. I had to learn how to change the kinds of food I ate and how I ate them. I learned to eat four to five 500-calorie meals during the day about three hours apart. Drinking water with every meal and in between helped fill me up without adding calories. Believe me, eating like this is tough when you're used to three square meals and a whole lot of snacking in between, but it's the only way to eat sensibly. With my workouts and active lifestyle, I burn about 3,000-3,500 calories a day for a caloric deficit of 500-1,000 calories and that's what you need to do, too.

All my life, people have told me, "Eat your fruits and vegetables." You know something? Those people are right because those foods are good fuel. My meals today consist of lean proteins, plenty of fruits and vegetables, and whole grains. That said, I will not deprive myself of something I crave every once in a while. I'll have some ice cream, cake, or pie now and then. I just remember not to overindulge, like I used to every day. It's okay to have these treats. Just watch your portions. Have a "cheat" meal once every couple of weeks. Not only will it make you feel like a normal human being, but you will probably also re-fire your metabolism. Sometimes giving your body something it hasn't had in a while will ramp up the weight loss to another level. Experiment and try new things to see what works for you.

Read Food Labels

Another important new habit I had to learn is to read food labels. Yeah, I know, it's tedious and boring, but so what? I wanted to lose weight and I knew changing my life was going to be hard work, so I committed myself to doing whatever would help me achieve my goal, even if it was tedious. Reading food labels helped me determine which foods to avoid and which to buy.

Ingredients on food labels are listed by weight with the top three containing most of the product. If one of those three is sugar, put it back! Also resist the temptation to buy foods with a high percentage of preservatives listed. There's an old saying: "If it rots, eat it." Or you might like this one better: "If it comes from a plant, eat it. If it's made in a plant, don't!"

Below is a reprint from the American Diabetes Association website of its guidelines for reading the nutritional elements of a food label:

Take a Closer Look at the Label

The information on the left side of the label provides total amounts of different nutrients per serving. To make wise food choices, check the total amounts for:

Using the information found in total amounts
Total amounts are shown in grams, abbreviated as g, or in milligrams, shown as mg. A gram is a very small amount and a milligram is one-thousandth of that. For example, a nickel weighs about 5 grams. So does a teaspoonful of margarine. Compare labels of similar foods. For example, choose the product with a smaller amount of saturated fat, cholesterol, and sodium and try to select foods with more fiber.

Calories
If you are trying to lose or maintain your weight, the number of calories you eat counts. To lose weight you need to eat fewer calories than your body burns. You can use the labels to compare similar products and determine which contains fewer calories. To find out how many calories you need each day, talk with your dietitian or certified diabetes educator.

Total Fat
Total fat tells you how much fat is in a food per serving. It includes fats that are good for you such as mono and polyunsaturated fats, and fats that are not so good such as saturated and trans fats. Mono and polyunsaturated fats can help to lower your blood cholesterol and protect your heart. Saturated and trans fat can raise your blood cholesterol and increase your risk of heart disease. The cholesterol in food may also increase your blood cholesterol. Learn more about specific types of fat.

Fat is calorie-dense. Per gram, it has more than twice the calories of carbohydrate or protein. Although some types of fats, such as mono and polyunsaturated fats, are healthy, it is still important to pay attention to the overall number of calories that you consume to maintain a healthy weight. If you are trying to lose weight, you'll still want to limit the amount of fat you eat. That's where the food label comes in handy.

Sodium

Sodium does not affect blood glucose levels. However, many people eat much more sodium than they need. Table salt is very high in sodium. You might hear people use "sodium" in lieu of "table salt," or vice versa.

With many foods, you can taste how salty they are, such as pickles or bacon. But there is also hidden salt in many foods, like cheeses, salad dressings, canned soups and other packaged foods. Reading labels can help you compare the sodium in different foods. You can also try using herbs and spices in your cooking instead of adding salt. Adults should aim for less than 2400 mg per day. If you have high blood pressure, it may be helpful to eat less.

Total Carbohydrate

If you are carbohydrate counting, the food label can provide you with the information you need for meal planning. Look at the grams of total carbohydrate, rather than the grams of sugar. Total carbohydrate on the label includes sugar, complex carbohydrate, and fiber. If you look only at the sugar number, you may end up excluding nutritious foods such as fruits and milks thinking they are too high in sugar. You might also overeat foods such as cereals and grains that have no natural or added sugar, but do contain a lot of carbohydrate.

The grams of sugar and fiber are counted as part of the grams of total carbohydrate. If a food has 5 grams or more fiber in a serving, subtract the fiber grams from the total grams of carbohydrate for a more accurate estimate of the carbohydrate content.

Fiber

Fiber is part of plant foods that is not digested. Dried beans such as kidney or pinto beans, fruits, vegetables and grains are all good sources of fiber. The recommendation is to eat 25-30 grams of fiber per day. People with diabetes need the same amount of fiber as everyone else.

Sugar alcohols

Sugar alcohols (also known as polyols) include sorbitol, xylitol and mannitol, and have fewer calories than sugars and starches. Use of sugar alcohols in a product does not necessarily mean the product is low in carbohydrate or calories. And, just because a package says "sugar-free" on the outside, that does not mean that it is calorie or carbohydrate-free. Always remember to check the label for the grams of carbohydrate and calories.

List of Ingredients

Ingredients are listed in descending order by weight, meaning the first ingredient makes up the largest proportion of the food. Check the ingredient list to spot things you'd like to avoid, such as coconut oil or palm oil, which are high in saturated fat. Also try to avoid hydrogenated oils that are high in trans fat. They are not listed by total amount on the label, but you can choose foods that don't list hydrogenated or partially hydrogenated oil in the ingredient list.

The ingredient list is also a good place to look for heart-healthy ingredients such as soy; monounsaturated fats such as olive, canola or peanut oils; or whole grains, like whole wheat flour and oats.

At this point you may be thinking, "Steve, I just can't do everything you're asking!" All I can say to that is if I could do it, anyone can. Remember, I have to manage my time because I have very little of it to go around, but I made time—it was that simple. If I didn't, I would've died too soon.

None of this is easy. Old habits die hard, but I continually remind myself of all those great American values I discussed earlier so that I'll keep those old habits at bay. Remember, if a fifty-one year old janitor can change what he eats and how he eats, so can you.

PART FOUR

❖◆◆◆

ENJOYING LIFE LIBERTY AND HAPPINESS

*We hold these truths to be self-evident, that all men are created equal,
that they are endowed by their Creator with certain
unalienable Rights that among these are Life, Liberty
and the pursuit of Happiness.*

~ Declaration of Independence

12

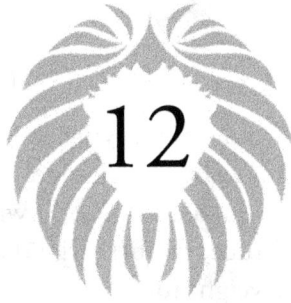

REAPING THE REWARDS

Sow an act and you reap a habit. Sow a habit and you reap a character.
Sow a character and you reap a destiny.

~ Charles Reade

◇◆◇◆

For the first time in a long time I'm a happy man. I lost a lot of what was bad in me and only some of it was weight. I gained new friends and experienced miraculous transformations in my life. It's as if I pulled down the zipper of my peasant body and roared out into a whole new world as a robust and powerful king. Writing this book is but one expression of that new-found freedom. Here are some others:

Appreciating the Little Things

I love this new body of mine because being in shape again just makes everything easier. I can tie my shoes, wash myself properly, and dry off using only one towel! I can trim my own toenails, wear jeans, and buckle a belt. I can now do so many things that others take for granted.

Banishing Fears

I've lived fifty-two years, most of them being afraid. I've disappointed many people in my life because of fear and I'm tired of it. Now I feel free and empowered to start doing things that take me out of my comfort zone where I am not in control of my destiny, like fly in an airplane, or take a tram ride. Sounds simple, but I refused to do these things before.

It's time to grow up. It's time to shake off the fear. There's a verse in I Corinthians that says, "When I was a child, I spoke as a child, I understood as a child, I thought as a child: but when I became a man, I put away childish things." Obesity has been put away. Now fear must fall, and it has.

71

Paying it Forward

My greatest fear was that I would die leaving my story forever buried, and I couldn't let that happen. I want to be a role model to as many people as I can—people like me who are hungry for a change. So I wrote a book and am becoming a mentor to others, like Bruce, my best friend since grade school who has been trying to get me to lose weight for years.

We always talked about playing a lot of golf when we retired, but Bruce truly thought I was going to be an invalid wheeling around in a chair instead of walking around a golf course. Now he says my transformation is the single most amazing thing he's ever witnessed in his life, but he was still not willing to undergo a makeover of his own.

Bruce aged a lot during his eight years as a high school athletic and activities director. Throughout that time, he always weighed in around 250 pounds, never getting any bigger but never losing anything either. Moreover, the stress and weight issues led to heart and digestive problems.

After he retired, he took a teaching job at a Christian school in North Carolina, but he wasn't in good enough shape, physically or mentally, to take on a full class load. He resigned, went home, and called me up. "I want to change my lifestyle, Steve," he said. "Then maybe I can be in shape to try the teaching thing again later." Bruce wanted me to be his accountability partner and show him the way, so I told him everything I'm telling you in this book. I also told him to check with his doctor first because of his health problems.

I told Bruce that the two most important things to do right away were to keep a lifestyle journal and to have someone hold him accountable. So he began to journal what he ate and how he exercised. He shows me his journal once a week, just like I did with Kelly. To date, he has taken off forty-five pounds and I'm sure he'll meet his weight goal very soon. He's confident that we can enjoy our retirement together and he can go back to teaching if he wants.

Preparing for Publicity with a Purpose

When I reached 228 pounds, Kelly contacted a local news station to tell them my story. I had my moment of fame on the *Healthy Living* segment of the six o'clock news. You can watch it at LionUnleashed.com. I agreed to the interview because I wanted to tell everyone that Kelly was the reason behind my entire life change, but she wanted absolutely no credit. In fact, she keeps telling me I am the one who did all the work, not her.

I'm glad I did the interview because a very sweet lady happened to see it and called to tell me that I saved her life. She said she was at the end of her rope when she saw me and that I encouraged her to get a grip on her life. Shortly after, I received this thank you note:

> *Steve,*
>
> *Just want to thank you again for literally saving my life. Thank you for keeping after that stubborn Tribune editor when he wouldn't publish your letter. Your wonderful persistence gave me the courage to change my life. You were so very nice on the phone that I felt like I was talking to a long-time friend. Hope to see you at TuDor!!!   -- Sandy*

Who knows how many other lives were touched by seeing my story on the news or reading my letter to the editor in our local paper, *The Tribune*. Who knows how many I'll impact with this book? I do know I've been able to touch some within my own circle of family and friends. One friend who is still working on her weight loss told me, "Steve I'm so proud of you. Every time I see you, I get more and more motivated."

I don't just want to look good. I want to inspire you to reach your own lifestyle and weight goals. I know you want to. You just need your own Kelly. She didn't merely offer me an outstretched hand and a kind smile. I only saw her once a week at most, but she inspired me by calling me out, equipping me, and continually believing I could do it. That's what I want to be to you.

Looking HOT

One day before my weight loss, with the help of a footstool, I rode a bike. I was pretty proud of myself until I turned back to see Bruce rolling on the ground with laughter: "You look like a golf ball sitting on a tee!"

Ha! That *was* me ... a big golf ball sitting on a tee. Nowadays, great-looking gals at work turn their heads and sweetly whisper, "Steve, if you get any hotter I'm not going to be able to stand it!" Now that's better.

Looking *hot* was not the goal of this lifestyle change. It really wasn't, but I have to admit that my ego is stroked when I wear jeans to work and hear "We see what you're wearing and we like what we see!" The two lady teachers who make comments like these have been my biggest cheerleaders on the job, and I'm glad to be able to give them some eye candy in return.

Kelly and Tina aren't satisfied with mere compliments. They want to see a fairy tale ending to this story, so they keep trying to fix me up with female companionship. I love them both to death, bless their hearts, but I just can't bring someone into the middle of my family problems. It wouldn't be fair to the not-so-lucky lady. My dear friends want to see children in this fairy tale, too. I'm pretty sure that's one miracle that their scientific skills cannot produce. But I guess anything is possible.

Even the photographer that I contracted to take some good *after* shots of me is a hopeful romantic. "Don't be surprised if you see some of your photos on the Internet because I'm going to post them," he said. "That will surely get you some phone calls!" It feels great when complete strangers compliment me on this hard-won achievement.

Being a Better Provider

I may feel like I can carry the world on my shoulders; but in reality, I know I can't, so I have to be realistic and settle with carrying my mom to the shower. It's a bittersweet arrangement. I get stronger as my parents get weaker, but that's the way God intended it. He always provides what we need, and He knew I needed strength, both physical and mental to take care of them to the end—and that's what I intend to do.

Preparing to Play

Climbing the stairs at work is sure a lot easier now. Heck, I might work a few more years. *Not!* This custodian will hang up his broom forever very soon. I plan on playing golf—a lot of golf. And since I've conquered my fear of flying, I'll fly all over the country to play, maybe even go to Scotland one day—another dream that will come true.

In the meantime, I'm having a blast relearning how to swing. Just the other day, when the sun was behind me, I reached back to take a lofty swing and there was my shadow staring back at me. I don't recall ever seeing my shadow there before. I laughed so hard, I missed the ball! That would've been funny once, but I did it two more times in a row. I saw my physique in a whole new light that day. It really was a brand new me!

By the time I retire, I'll have a new backswing and a better game. Maybe I'll become a starter on a golf course to supplement my retirement. That would be a pretty cool job. I probably won't become a Walmart greeter, though, in case you were wondering.

Playing the Back Six

My nephew J.D. told me that while he was playing basketball at the park, there was on "old guy" playing with them who was pretty good.

"How old was this old guy?" I asked.

"Forty," he said.

"Forty? I'm fifty-one! If forty is old, what does that make me?"

J.D. calmly replied, "Well Uncle Steve, you're definitely on the back nine of life."

While I understand what he meant, I have to disagree. It's more like the back six. I definitely have more years behind me than ahead of me, but God has a plan for those years. God heals people so He will get the credit and so that His purposes will be fulfilled. I believe God healed me so I can help you achieve freedom from the disadvantages of the handicap of obesity, but that would be an empty pursuit if I don't also tell you that God wants to call you to Him so He can give you freedom forever with Him in eternity.

For forty years, I lived like I wanted to, not the way He wanted me to. You see, I didn't believe I needed Jesus to save me from anything. I believed I was a good person and did good things, but compared to God, the Bible says I'm not good at all. I don't want my old degenerative life or body anymore. I want a new life and I have one through Jesus Christ, who paid the price for my sinful nature. Now I trust Him to guide my steps in the future as He did in the past year and a half. Of course, as a fellow American, you don't have to believe in anything or anybody, but I sure hope you'll consider starting your new life with Jesus rather than without Him.

13

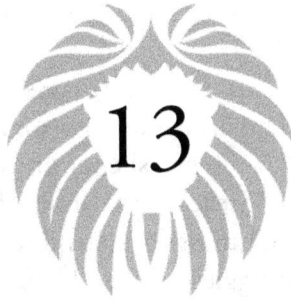

MAINTAIN YOUR WEIGHT LOSS

You have failed only when you quit trying.
Until then, you're still in the act of progression.
So, never quit trying and you'll never be a failure.

~ Tommy Kelley

◆◆◇◇

"Look, there's a stranger in the house!" My mom says. She witnessed every yo-*yo*-yo, but never gave up on me. She is now so proud of my achievement. But she regularly warns me, in her own sweet way, that if I don't watch out the weight will creep back up on me. As always, she's right. At times I have gained enough for people to notice, but I gave her my word this time on the Holy Bible that I'm not going back, ever, to my former lifestyle.

That said, I battle to maintain my weight every day. It's not easy. I have gained ten to fifteen pounds several times while writing this book. The major culprits are my biggest weaknesses—junk food and lack of journaling. I've learned that when I fall, I have to take the following immediate action:

- First, I start journaling again, which forces me to see how much junk I'm eating.

- Second, I confess my lack of self-discipline to my support team on my Spark People blog at SparkPeople.com and ask them to make me accountable again. My teammates on that site understand setbacks and we uplift each other. I also call Bruce and we mentor each other. I can't do this alone and you probably can't either, which is why you must surround yourself with a support system.

- Finally, I stop at TuDor to get a pat on the back or a kind word from the gang there and then I walk over to the gym to work out.

My greatest fear is that I'll put all that excess cargo back on. I fear for my health and I fear bringing embarrassment to everyone who stuck out their necks for me, especially Kelly, but even she reminds me that my accountability must be to Someone higher: "Steve, make yourself accountable to God," she wrote in a note. "With Him all things are possible." I have faith that God will see me through these daily struggles because He said He would.

14

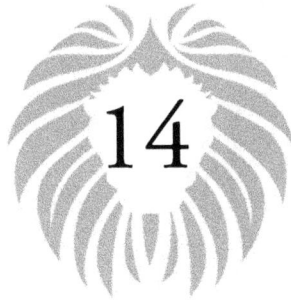

FINAL THOUGHTS

Sometimes in the winds of change we find our true direction.

~ Anonymous

◇◆◇◆◇

As you can probably tell by now, I really am about as average as you can imagine. As I embark on the last stretch of my life journey, I can't be afraid to roar about what is possible or my story will fade away and you might fade away with it. Maybe someone else will tell a similar story, but this one was given for me to tell. From the bottom of my heart, I hope my story has helped you.

Until now I've never taken my wall down as I have in these pages. I do not mean to boast or sound arrogant in any way, but I am very pleased and proud of what I've accomplished. So before I close, I'm going to take one last chance to roar: "Hello world; look at me now, I've lost 160 pounds. I'm one hot fifty-two year old man. And I feel great!"

Okay, that's it. I'm putting my wall back up now, hanging up the no trespassing sign, and I'm outta here!

EPILOGUE

◈◈◈

Sorry, but I have to take the no trespassing sign down again for a brief moment. I need to share with you that during the editing of this book, I lost my brother due to complications from alcoholism. I *loved* my brother but I was angry with him and didn't *like* him very much during the several years he lived with me and my parents. During the year and a half I was going through my transformation, he made things very difficult. I don't know if you've ever had an alcoholic in your family, but I'm sure many of you have. I have tried very hard not to be negative or judgmental in this book, but some of that may come out now because the situation has resolved itself.

My brother was unemployed for the last eight years of his life and he had no transportation of his own. My dad funded his habits. He lived in the basement of our house. All he did was drink beer and smoke cigarettes. There were many arguments between the two of them until my dad began to have short-term memory problems. The dementia that runs in his family finally began to manifest itself. Seeing this happen, I wanted my brother to leave my dad alone so I gave him money to keep him from bothering Dad. He constantly begged me to drive him to the corner store to get his supplies … every day. I told him I'd do it every other day, but that didn't last too long. His addictions caused a daily need for the stuff. So soon I was not only paying for it, I was driving him to get it. When I'd argue and refuse, he'd complain to Dad and Dad would beg me to take him. All I wanted was peace, so I just started buying the stuff when I was out. Some of you may call me an enabler; but unless you've dealt with dementia and alcoholism under the same roof, I don't think you would be able to understand.

It was brutal most of the time. There I was in the middle of it trying to change my life and there he was … constantly arguing even though he was getting his stuff. Alcoholics regularly complain and are very selfish people. This caused great stress in my life, but I stayed the course. I don't think I can fully explain just how difficult the situation turned out to be. The more my brother deteriorated, the meaner he became. We tried so hard to get him help, but he refused to go to the hospital or see a doctor. He was watching me change and overcome right before his eyes, and in one of his better moments he even told me he was proud of me. He said, "I wish I could do what you're doing but I just can't. I need it, brother!"

Finally it all caught up with him. He began vomiting pure blood. We called 911 and he was rushed to the hospital where he died of massive internal bleeding right in front of me, my sister, and my nephew … a sad ending to a wasted life.

Looking back I now realize that I actually learned a lot from my brother. I learned what happens when you make wrong choices and waste your life. My brother always used to tell me, "Steve, you can't preach to me about my habits. Look at you. You're eating your way to an early grave. You do it your way and I'll do it mine!" Looking back, I see that he was right. I'd always hoped that if he saw me change my life, he would wake up to the fact that it could be done, like it did with Bruce. Sadly it did not.

I witnessed firsthand what making wrong choices can do to a person; and after seeing that, it has further strengthened my resolve to *never* go back again. Maybe alcoholism and obesity aren't the same, but don't you agree that either way you are shortening your life? So I'd like to thank my brother for helping me see that. Through his death he empowered me even more.

◇◈◈◇

In part two of this epilogue, I've discovered that writing a book and having it published and distributed are totally different things. There's a lot of time between the two … a lot. I started writing this book as a novice in April of 2008. When I submitted the first draft of the manuscript to my publisher, it was October of 2008, but personal setbacks and trials got in the way for her as much as it did for me at various stages throughout this process. But we stuck it out together and after many drafts and much work and prayer, it is now in your hands.

I'm a very patient man; GOD blessed me with that quality. I'm so very thankful to my publisher/ghostwriter, for taking on my project. She took my amateur chicken scratch and turned it into this work of art you've just read. I've come to trust her as a friend, even though we have never personally met. This project was completed via the internet and a couple of phone calls.

I said all that because many things have happened to me since the death of my brother in January of 2009. Most of the book was finished long before that date. I want to be totally honest with you, my readers, because you have to know that I'm just like you, an ordinary person with ordinary problems. I'm not some Superman who has all the right answers or does all the right things.

After my brother passed away, things were okay for the longest time. But beginning in December of 2009, I began to have many personal problems that got me way off track. Some I'll not get into right now because they're not resolved. But I'll share one of them with you. My dad was diagnosed with male breast cancer. He had a radical mastectomy on January 1, 2010. With his dementia I was at a loss on what to do. It was decided by our family to not put him through chemotherapy or radiation. The pathology report had it as grade II cancer. That means there is a slight risk of spread. We decided not to put him through living hell and put it all in God's hands.

Well, me being me fell back into some old familiar behaviors. I put 60 pounds back on between December of 2009 and March of 2010. I got back up to 250 pounds from my low of 190. I used my personal problems as excuses to begin my bad habits again. You have to know that because I'm not here to lie to you. It's so easy to get your focus off God and fail miserably.

This is where God intervened yet again and led me to some new people to help get me back on track. Enter Dr. John Mistretta and Butch Temnick.

Dr. Mistretta is my chiropractor and very good friend. I asked him to read the manuscript and give me a blurb for the book. He did that and more. He lined up a speaking engagement for me at a local school to give a talk about my weight loss and life-style change. He also wants to do more of these to help me push the book as well as his business. You scratch my back, I'll scratch yours kind of deal. I'm not a public speaker but he said doing things like that would help me "practice what I preach" and keep me focused and on track. I was well received and now I have to stay on point with my eating and exercise.

Butch Temnick came into my life through my gym, Global Health and Fitness. He's known as Mr. Wellness. He's a certified fitness expert, nutritionist, and teacher of a program called Transitions Lifestyle System. I signed up for his 12-week course that began in April of 2010. It's based on the low glycemic index and I'm learning how to eat right again. Emotional eating has always been my downfall and this program is just what I needed at this point in my life. It's not that far away from what I was doing before. It's just a little tweak of concentrating on the kinds of foods that don't cause a spike in your blood sugar. Staying away from sugar and processed foods. My plan was right; it just needed a little tweak. I've said many times that you need to make a change here and there to trick your body. This was my new trick. I'm in the middle of the program as of this writing and I'm back down to 210 pounds and have 20 more to go to get to my 190-pound goal.

Butch is a breath of fresh air and I believe God caused our paths to cross. His enthusiasm is boundless and it's rubbed off on me. I'm back on fire again and more focused than ever.

Things happen in all of our lives that can cause us to falter and fail. If you learn nothing else from this book, please see how my faith in God failed me many times, but HE did not. HE tested me and I failed. But He loved me so much; he put me back on track by increasing my support system.

People are placed into our lives by God all the time. But, we have to see His hand is the guiding hand, not those people. As much as I deeply care for all of the new people in my life, I have to always remember who really deserves the credit here. People tell me I deserve the credit because I did the work. Well, I beg to differ. I wouldn't have done the work had those people not come into my life. And even more than that … those people wouldn't have come into my life had God not ordained it. So the credit here once again goes to my Lord and Savior, Jesus Christ.

◆◆◆◆

Note from the Publisher

In this third part of the Epilogue, I must let readers know about the man behind the lion as I know him. I have never met such a humble, gentle, patient, and decent man as Stephen. His passion to help people live a healthier, happier life as God intended for them to live is genuine. His empathy for others' trials is also genuine because he has faced so many himself. He is not judgmental, but understanding and supportive. I have seen God's providence in his transformed life and in the process of getting this book written and published. God would not let the project die. He has great plans for Stephen and the hundreds, if not thousands, of lives who will be touched by him and his lion that is now, finally, unleashed!

APPENDIX

APPENDIX A

Resources

Below are web sites and resources that I've personally used while losing and maintaining weight. They will provide a starting point as you begin to study about and design your own weight-loss program. These same resources and others are frequently updated at **lionunleashed.com**.

Sparkpeople at **sparkpeople.com** is a free weight-loss community with people just like us. You can e-mail, blog, and chat with experts and ordinary people 24/7. Great advice, diet plans, exercise tips, and videos guide you. I highly recommend this web site.

Dick's Sporting Goods at **DicksSportingGoods.com** is an excellent place to find workout apparel, stability balls, heart rate monitors, workout shoes, etc. Any sporting goods store will be a great place for you to find the right workout equipment and apparel.

GNC or General Nutrition Centers at **gnc.com** is one of many nutrition sites where you can buy vitamins, protein shake mixes, amino acid powders, and even workout equipment. I have found the customer service reps to be very knowledgeable, so feel free to ask questions.

Global Health and Fitness at **globalfitnesswarren.com** is my gym. You need to find a gym and make it your home away from home.

Burn the Fat: Feed the Muscle at **TheFatBurnFiles.com** is a paid membership web site run by fitness and nutrition expert, Tom Venuto. It has diet and exercise plans galore and a chat community. Advice of all kinds abounds here as well as support from people battling to lose weight and build a healthier body. This is a great resource if you want to spend a little money, and I mean *a little money*. It's a modest investment for all you get in return.

Fitness experts like Tom Venuto and those listed below sell e-books on training techniques with money back guarantees. I have purchased their basic programs and interacted with them on their forums. I still implement many of their tips and believe these experts really want to help people live healthier lives:

- Darin Steen, **FatLossLifestyle.com**

- Jillian Michaels, **jillianmichaels.com**

- Jon Benson, **jonbenson.com**

YouTube at **youtube.com** hosts exercise video demonstrations by the experts listed above. This is where I learned how to do a lot of my body weight and stability ball workouts. Be careful, though. Anyone can post a video on YouTube and anyone does. Search only for known fitness experts as you learn how to perform exercises correctly.

APPENDIX B

My Workout Regimen

I am not a fitness expert, so please check with your doctor and/or a certified fitness trainer before starting any exercise program. My workout regimen is provided only for reference purposes.

Since joining a gym, I have been working out seven days a week—six days at the gym plus a weekly visit at TuDor. Working out is all about progressing and graduating. You progress in time and duration (such as walking to running) and graduate in the amount of weight and the type of machine you use.

For the first year or so, every progression and graduation was really hard work. I left feeling so sore, but the soreness also made me feel so good because the endorphins the brain produces during a workout soothed me with a natural high. It was just icing on the cake as the pounds rolled off.

After mastering the simpler exercises, I started weight training on the Nautilus equipment, which does not use free weights. After several weeks, I graduated to the Hammer strength equipment, which is a combination of machine weights and free weights. The Hammer equipment stabilizes the free weight equally, so I never have to worry about dropping it. Then I moved up to free weights alone. Lifting free weights forces you to do the stabilizing, which means you're using bigger muscles to lift the weight and smaller muscles to stabilize the weight equally. Ask a trainer to explain this to you before you try free weights on your own or you could easily hurt yourself.

Each day includes some form of cardio machine, such as the elliptical machine, recumbent stationary bike, treadmill, and stair climber. Monday, Wednesday and Friday are weight training days in addition to cardio training. I do my upper body workout Monday and Friday and lower body on Wednesday because my muscles need those alternate days off to recover.

It's a sore subject in the fitness industry—steady-state cardio. Many people don't like it. They think it's boring and really doesn't help. I happen to disagree. It worked for me because it was one of those change-ups I talked about. Any time I changed my workout routine, I got results. And that's all that really matters, right?

Throughout my weight loss journey, I educated myself online, in the library, and by talking to professionals about fitness and nutrition. Eventually I discovered that all roads lead to the same training principle; that is, interval training—a series of short intense sprints of exercise followed by longer rest periods. Interval training is about exercising your heart by getting the heart rate up very high during the short bursts and getting it back down during the longer recovery period, so you have to gradually work up to it. You can't do this as a beginner.

I spoke to Kelly at Tudor as well as the staff at Global about interval training, and they all agreed that it was the best way to increase muscle mass and ramp up my metabolism to maximum levels. So I tried it and it worked! The more muscle I put on, the more my metabolism increased because my body needed to burn more calories throughout the day just to sustain itself. This is called the "after burn" effect, technically known as Exercise Post Oxygen Consumption or EPOC. Keep in mind that you have to gradually work your way up to interval training. It took several months after I first started walking before my body was ready for exercise this vigorous. The first couple of weeks were really tough leaving my body groaning with exhaustion. You know ... that naturally high, groaning kind of exhaustion.

Today, interval training is an integral part of my overall exercise plan in which I alternate interval training days with steady-state cardio days. Steady-state cardio gets my heart rate up to 85% of its maximum and keeps it there for the entire session. It's important to ask your doctor what your maximum heart rate should be while exercising. Also invest in a good quality heart rate monitor. I chose the Polar brand, which offers several models to fit your style.

With steady-state cardio, I burn calories only during the workout, but during interval training, I'm burning calories well after I leave the gym. Even so, it's still good to do both of these types of cardio for that "change-up" effect. Remember, the key is to fool your body by not letting it get used to the same routine. Changing-up also keeps your exercise from becoming boring. It adds new challenges and spice to your workout.

Around this time, I asked Bill what was the biggest mistake we gym rats make. He answered, "Doing the same workout over and over again. When I work out, I do different exercises every time because the body gets used to the same old routine and when that happens, it will not respond!" Kelly agreed. By this time I was in tune with how my body reacted to various workout regimens, so I created my own workout plan incorporating different machines on different days. When I hit a plateau I knew how to do my own tweaking. Sometimes that meant just a slight change in the intensity or duration of an exercise; and when I did that … ***bam***. I was off and running again, pushing the limits of my physical abilities.

&#x03;

Before I leave for the gym, I plan on paper the machines I'll use, how much weight I'll start with and how many sets I'll do. Below is a typical weight-day workout for me.

Please do not incorporate this routine into your own training. I only provide it as an example of how to prepare an interval workout. If possible, create your own plan with a personal trainer.

My Typical Workout Plan for the Day

Today, I'll work out on six Nautilus machines:

- Seated shoulder press
- Seated row machine
- Seated chest press with the same routine
- Seated biceps curling machine
- Incline chest press machine
- Triceps pull down machine

On each machine I'll do:

	1st Set	2nd Set	3rd Set	4th Set
	rest 30 sec	rest 30 sec	rest 30 sec	
Weight:	90	100	110	120
Repetitions	10	10	10	10

The next day that I work on my upper body, I do this same six-machine routine, but I'll either up the weight and use less sets and reps or lower the weight and use more sets and reps. That's how I change it up.

Every day is cardio day. On lifting days I do interval cardio, and on non-lifting days I do steady-state cardio by working out on either the bike, the elliptical, the treadmill, or stair climber. If I have a lot of energy I'll do two machines, but it's not necessary.

Here's a typical example of how I've tweaked the recumbent stationary bike to fit my interval cardio needs:

I set the timer to nineteen minutes on level 16. Each machine has levels of difficulty ranging from 1-20. All the machines have pre-set programs or you can set your own. I set mine by selecting "manual." This way I control my own sprint and recovery paces.

I warm up for the first five minutes at a moderate pace. There's no warm-up button. I just proceed at a moderate pace.

Then I peddle as fast as I can for a thirty-second sprint and follow that with a sixty-second slower paced recovery period. I do ten of these sets, which takes me through the nineteen minutes.

I cool down for three minutes (all the machines have a mandatory three to five minute cool down period) making it a vigorous twenty-two minute workout.

I enjoy working out on a different cardio machine every day because I learned the hard way that familiarity with one not only slowed down my progress, it made exercising a bore—and as I said earlier, exercise should never be boring.

APPENDIX C

Appendix C starts on the next page.

APPENDIX C

Date: 1-05-08	Date: 1-06-08	Date: 1-07-08
Breakfast	**Breakfast**	**Breakfast**
· 1 slice whole grain whole wheat toast · 1 hardboiled egg · water Snack: 25 raw almonds and water	· 2 slices whole grain rye toast/almond butter · water Snack: 10 garlic and herb wheat thins and water	· 2 hardboiled eggs · 4 oz. can of tuna fish · water Snack: 25 raw walnuts and water
Lunch	**Lunch**	**Lunch**
· ¼ head raw cabbage · 3 carrots · 3 pickle cucumbers · 8 radishes · Protein shake · water Snack: 25 raw almonds and water	· 8 oz. baked pork loin · Bell pepper slices · side salad · water Snack: 6 mini wheat's biscuits and water	· 2 baked 8 oz. boneless chicken breast · side salad · water Snack: 10 garlic and herb wheat thins, cup of green tea, and water
Dinner	**Dinner**	**Dinner**
· Dinner salad · 12 oz. sirloin steak · Plain baked potato · water Snack: 25 raw almonds	· 3 Cajun chicken wings · 8 radishes · 3 carrots · ¼ head cabbage · 2 pickle cucumbers · water Snack: 10 garlic and herb wheat thins	· 4 oz. baked chicken breast · 2 Cajun chicken wings · 2 carrots · water Snack: 25 raw almonds and water
Exercise	**Exercise**	**Exercise**
Minutes: 135 · 30 min. on treadmill · 30 min. on bike · 30 min. on elliptical · Upper body lifting: · Seated chest press · Incline bench press · Seated shoulder press · 100 pounds-3 sets of 10 reps each.	Minutes: 100 Gym was closed today so I did crunches, planks, and push-ups on my stability ball at home, then I power walked 3 ½ miles in an hour at the middle school track.	Minutes: 100 · 45 min. on elliptical · Leg work with weights · Squats on smith machine · Seated leg press · Leg curls (thighs) · Front and rear lunges with 25 pound dumb bells.

Stephen's Daily Journal

Date: 1-08-08	Date: 1-09-08	Date: 1-10-08
Breakfast	**Breakfast**	**Breakfast**
· 8 mini wheat's biscuits with ¼ cup no fat milk · 1 slice whole grain rye · toast · water Snack: carrot and celery sticks and water	· 2 slices whole grain whole wheat toast · 2 hardboiled eggs · water Snack: protein bar and water	· 4 oz. can tuna fish · ¼ head of raw lettuce · 1 slice whole grain rye · water Snack: 25 raw almonds and water
Lunch	**Lunch**	**Lunch**
· 8 radishes · 4 pickle cucumbers · 2 carrots · ¼ head raw cabbage · water Snack: 25 raw walnuts and water	· 2 baked four oz. turkey breast cutlets · side salad · water Snack: protein shake and water	· 2 baked four oz. turkey breast cutlets · side salad · water Snack: protein shake and water
Dinner	**Dinner**	**Dinner**
· 12 oz. rib eye · Side salad · 2 slices of pumpernickel bread · Cup of green beans · water Snack: 25 raw almonds and water	· Chicken Caesar salad · No dressing...salt and pepper · 25 raw almonds · water Snack: 6 mini wheat biscuits and water	· Foot long turkey breast sub from Subway/ spinach and onions · water Snack: 25 raw almonds and water
Exercise	**Exercise**	**Exercise**
Minutes: 135 · 3 ½ mile power walk at track · 30 min. on elliptical · Upper body workout · Preacher curls: biceps · Hammer curls with dumb bells · Lat pull downs · Seated rows	Minutes: 100 · Triceps pull downs · Butterfly chest pulls · Assisted dips and pull-ups · 45 min. on elliptical	Minutes: 100 · Seated shoulder press · Seated chest press · Incline bench press · 60 min. on treadmill at 3 mph with 15 degree incline...very tough

APPENDIX D

Date_____   Date_____   Date_____

Breakfast	**Breakfast**	**Breakfast**
Snack:	Snack:	Snack:
Lunch	**Lunch**	**Lunch**
Snack:	Snack:	Snack:
Dinner	**Dinner**	**Dinner**
Snack:	Snack:	Snack:
Exercise	**Exercise**	**Exercise**
Minutes_____ Type:	Minutes_____ Type:	Minutes_____ Type:

My Daily Journal

Date_____   Date_____   Date_____

Breakfast	**Breakfast**	**Breakfast**
Snack:	Snack:	Snack:
Lunch	**Lunch**	**Lunch**
Snack:	Snack:	Snack:
Dinner	**Dinner**	**Dinner**
Snack:	Snack:	Snack:
Exercise	**Exercise**	**Exercise**
Minutes_____ Type:	Minutes_____ Type:	Minutes_____ Type:

Ask Stephen to Speak

Stephen speaks to small and large groups at hospitals, schools, Rotary Clubs, and anywhere people need to receive the motivation and knowledge that Stephen offers.

Ask Stephen to Be Your Personal Lifestyle Coach

Do you need someone to help you plan a lifestyle change and hold you accountable to that plan? Mentoring others is Stephen's passion and he would be honored to do that for his readers.

Order Books

Individual and bulk orders of *Lion Unleashed* can be ordered in paperback and e-reader formats at LionUnleashed.com and major online bookstores.

Follow Stephen's Blog

Ask Stephen questions and follow his triumphs and setbacks during the rest of his lifestyle change journey at

LIONUNLEASHED COM

◆◆◆◆

"Sometimes we go through life passing roads that we fail to realize are even there. Steve Hosaflook's *Lion Unleashed* is a street sign that points down the right path."

~ George Garrett - Principal of Neal Middle School in Fowler, Ohio

NOTES